THE COMPLETE
Wellbeing
Manual

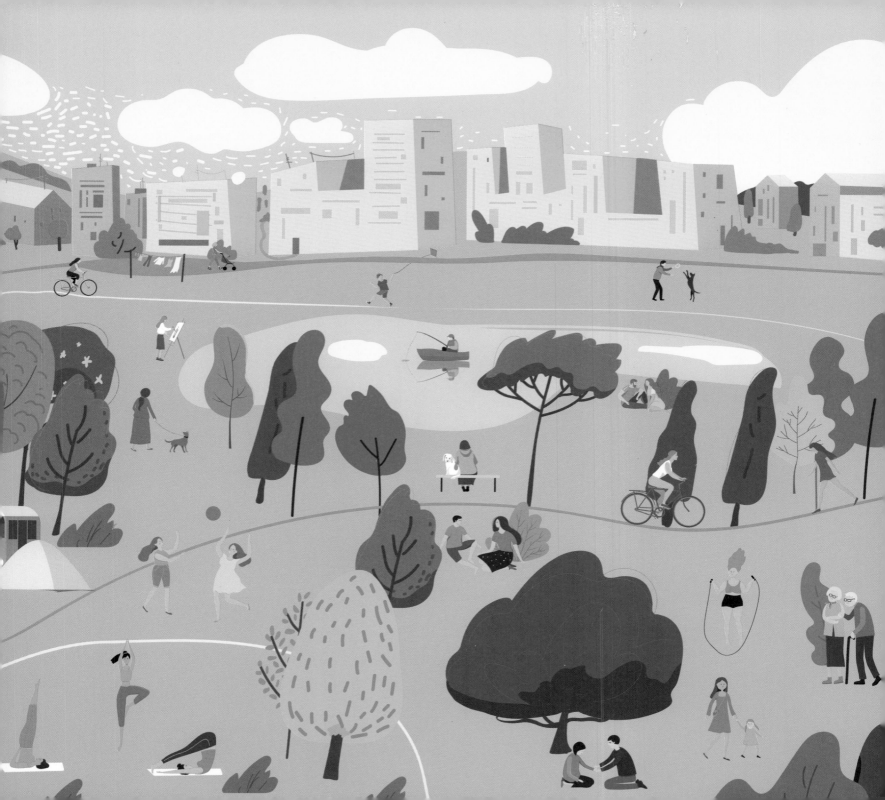

THE COMPLETE
Wellbeing
Manual

Your guide to an optimally healthy mind and body

EDITED BY EMMA VAN HINSBERGH
& FELICITY FORSTER

SIRIUS

CONTRIBUTORS: Jeff Archer, Christine Bailey, Eve Boggenpoel, Simone Bose, Sally Brown, Lisa Buckingham, Oliver Burkeman, Gemma Calvert, Rachel Chalmers, Larissa Chapman, Anita Chaudhuri, Samantha Clarke, Nigel Cumberland, Amy Dawson, Lizzy Dening, Lizzie Enfield, Helen Foster, Eva Gizowska, Lynda Gratton, Charlotte Haigh, Jessica Harris, Carly Hobbs, Liz Hollis, Abi Jackson, Angela Kennedy, Natalie Millman, Kim Morgan, Kristen Neff, Michele O'Connor, Chantelle Pattemo, Louise Pynem, Sam Rice, Andrew J. Scott, Heidi Scrimgeour, Sarah Sellens, Lily Smith, Rebecca Speechley, Cathy Struthers, Katy Sunnassee, Nolan Sunnassee, Suzy Walker, Mars Webb, Kim Willis, Wendy Green

SIRIUS

This edition published in 2022 by Sirius Publishing, a division of Arcturus Publishing Limited, 26/27 Bickels Yard, 151–153 Bermondsey Street, London SE1 3HA

Text, and images on pages 146–8, 150–1 and 232–5 © Kelsey Publishing Ltd 2022
Design © Arcturus Holdings Ltd 2022

All other images courtesy of Shutterstock

ISBN: 978-1-3988-0244-5
AD007321US

Printed in China

CONTENTS

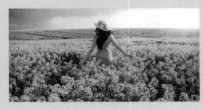

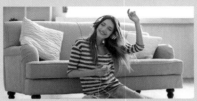

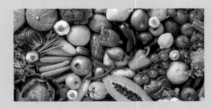

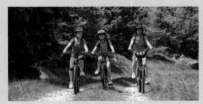

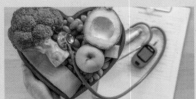

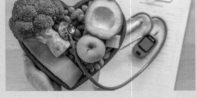

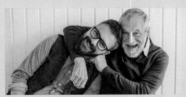

Introduction 6

Lifestyle 12

Free your mind 48

Eat well 92

Move your body 130

Health matters 164

Healthy aging 208

Planners 246
Index 252

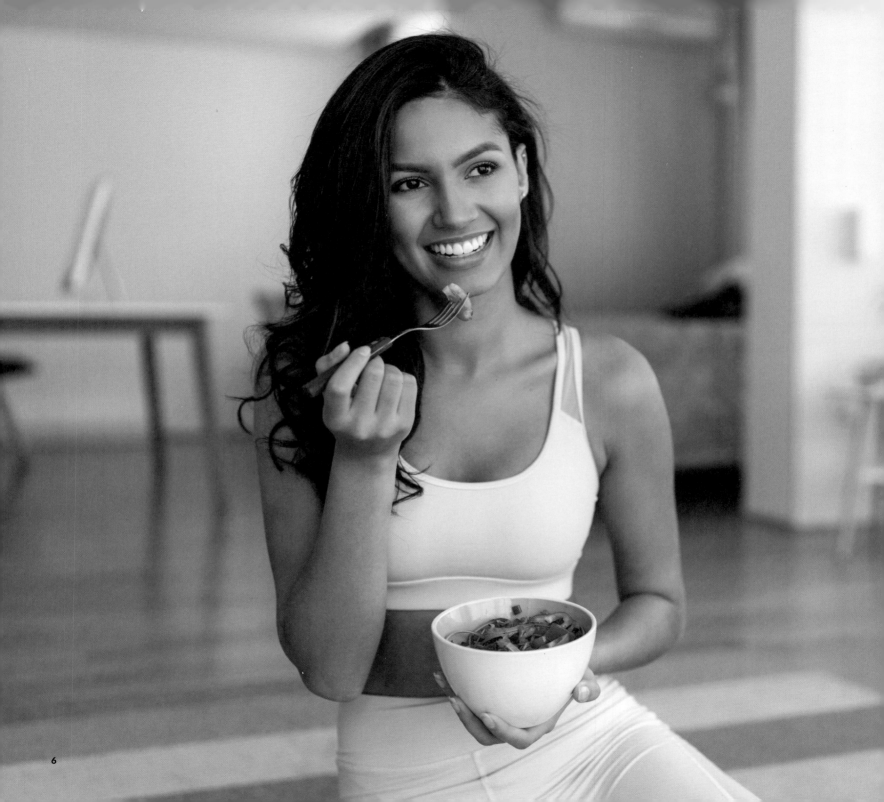

INTRODUCTION

Feeling healthy and happy is something we all aspire to, and no matter what stage of life we are at now, there is always room for a little improvement. This book is positively bursting with ideas for boosting your wellbeing, with chapters on lifestyle, mental health, nutrition, exercise, physical health, and aging. You can read it in any order—start from the beginning, or just dip in whenever you feel the need for a pick-me-up!

INTRODUCTION

Learning to look after your mental and physical wellbeing is one of the greatest gifts you can give yourself.

It's all too easy to carry on regardless, often unaware of what's really going on with our bodies or how certain situations might be affecting our health and happiness. But letting go of what you cannot change and making small and simple changes to your lifestyle, diet, and exercise can have a hugely positive impact on your life.

This handy book has everything you need to inspire you to make those changes and to bring balance and harmony into your life. Learn how to overhaul your lifestyle, banish stress, supercharge your diet, reach your fitness goals, and boost your vitality levels.

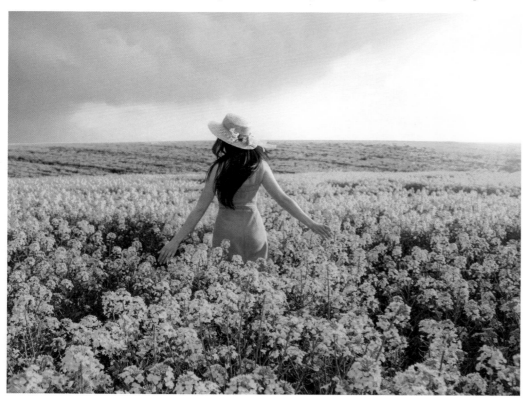

As you take your first steps on your journey toward health and wellbeing, it's a good idea to take a moment to think about the way in which you live now. Assessing your current lifestyle will really help before you start thinking about your wellbeing goals. Have a look at the table of questions on the page opposite, and begin by making some notes about your current lifestyle. Not only can this be a useful exercise in its own right, but it also means that in the future you can look back at your notes and see how much progress you've made.

Left: We can all benefit from improved health and wellbeing. Even small changes can make a huge difference. Not only will they make us feel physically healthier, but they will also reduce stress and give us a more positive outlook on life.

QUESTIONS TO CONSIDER

Here are a few questions to help you to think about your current lifestyle:

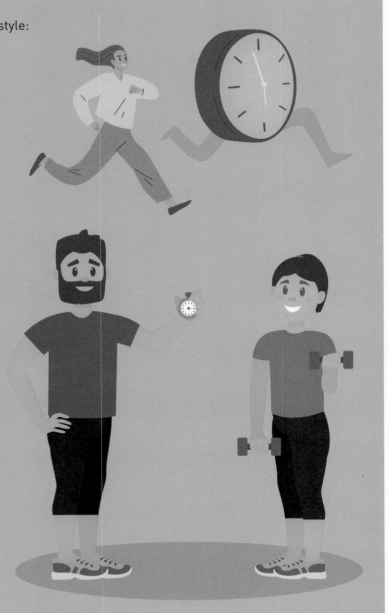

- How old are you and where are you now in your life? Are you working or retired? Do you have a spouse or partner? Do you have children? Do you live alone?

- How much free time do you have? Are you time-poor or do you have lots of spare time? How many free minutes or hours per day do you have? Do you take holidays?

- How do you feel on most days? Do you ever feel tired, anxious, depressed, or "wrung-out?" If you're working, would you say you have a good "work/life balance?" Do you enjoy your work?

- What is your living space like? Is your home chaotic or neat? Do you spend much time outdoors?

- What are your attitudes to food and nutrition? How many meals do you eat per day? Do you snack? Do you have any particular food preferences or allergies? Are you a meat-eater, vegetarian, vegan, or pescatarian? Do you have any food intolerances? Do you drink alcohol?

- What daily habits do you have? Are you an early riser or a night owl? Do you fall asleep easily? How many hours' sleep do you get per night? Do you smoke? Do you exercise regularly? How fit are you? What sort of exercise do you do, and for how long?

- What is your overall approach to health and wellbeing? Do you tend to take things as they come, or are you proactive and energetic in your quest for wellbeing? Do you have any particular health concerns right now?

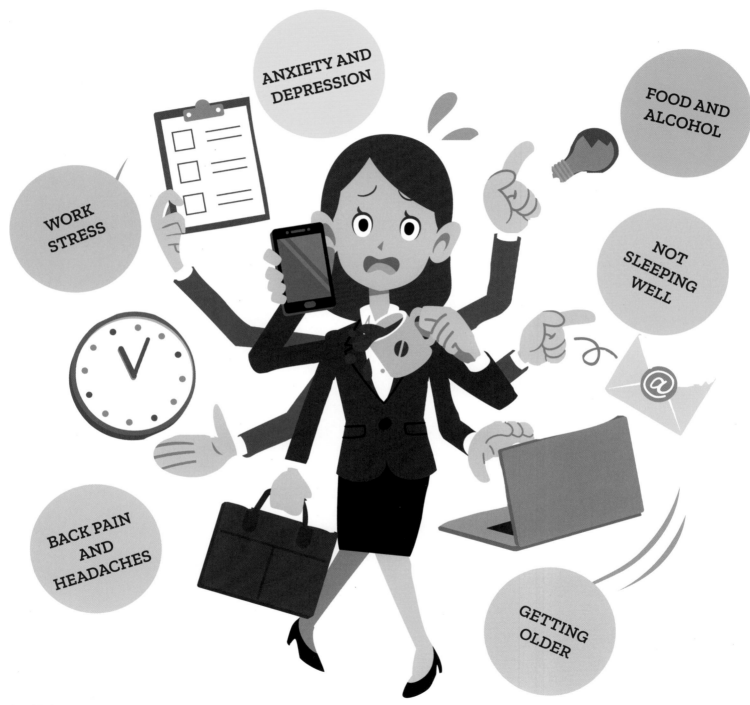

The way in which you live is affected by internal factors such as your physical health and state of mind, as well as external factors such as work and relationships. It is inextricably bound up with your mental wellbeing, nutrition, exercise, health, and aging—so it's important to think about all of these.

Whatever answers you give to the questions on page 9, there are almost certainly areas that you would like to improve, and this book provides plenty of ideas for doing just that. If you're looking to achieve a better work/life balance, eat more healthily, boost your immune system, help your hormones, improve your fitness, get a better night's sleep, lower your stress levels, or banish health niggles, you'll find it inside these pages. Use the book in whichever way works best for you. Dip into it whenever you need help or inspiration. If you find a piece of advice or health technique that resonates with you, practice it as long as it is helpful, then move on to something else when you need to.

Trust your instincts and your body. They know what's best for you.

Below: *Feeling better is within our control, and taking steps toward improving our wellbeing gives us a sense of purpose. Forest bathing can remind us of our connection with nature.*

BENEFITS OF HEALTH AND WELLBEING
- Boosts feelings of positivity and relaxation, and gives you a sense of purpose and control over your life.
- Improves your energy and productivity.
- Improves your mental health and resilience, and lowers the impact of stress, anxiety, and depression.
- Strengthens your muscles, helps you to feel fitter and more flexible, reduces aches and pains, lowers your blood pressure, improves the health of your heart, and lowers your risk of diabetes.
- Improves the quality of your sleep.
- Boosts immunity and improves your eating and drinking habits.
- Improves your social interactions.
- Helps you to live a longer, happier, and healthier life, and allows you to be the best person you can be.

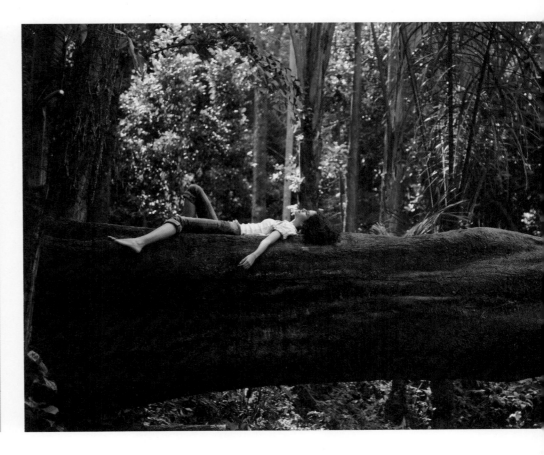

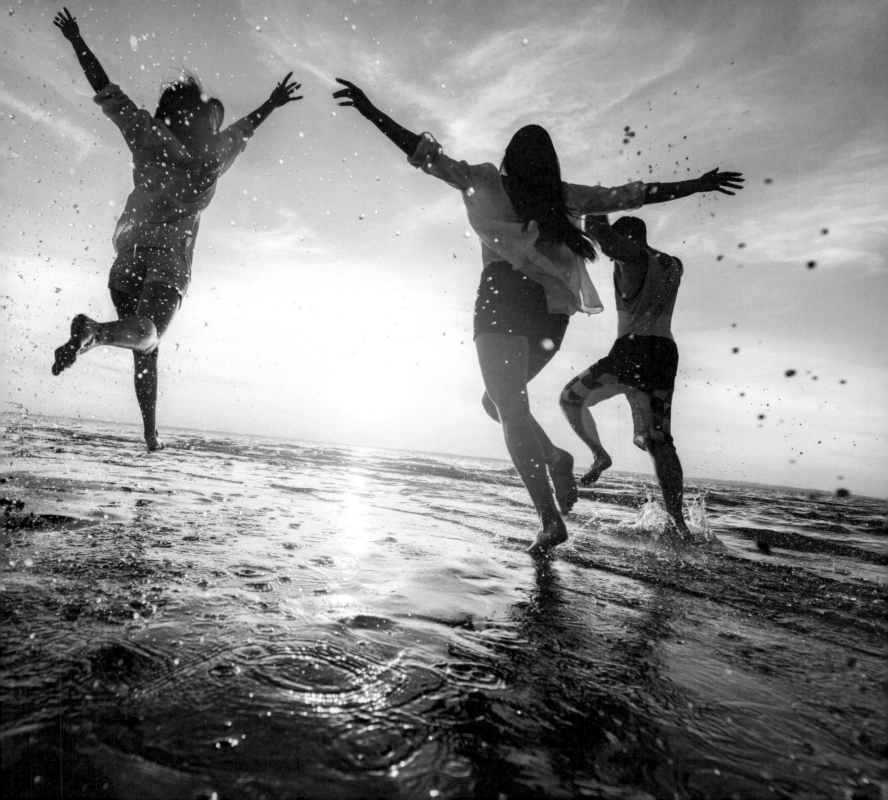

1
LIFESTYLE

Life can be demanding, and finding that sweet spot between work, family, relationships, and other commitments can often be a serious juggling act. This chapter shows how to achieve it, from decluttering your environment and learning breathwork and stress-busting solutions, to making friends, finding a job you love, and creating a happier work/life balance.

DECLUTTER YOUR ENVIRONMENT

There are many ways to spring-clean your health. And, it turns out, detoxing your environment can have a huge impact on your inner wellbeing.

Clearing out your clutter can be liberating, and the science is stacking up to prove it can have tangible mental health benefits, making you happier and more productive. It can even improve your diet. "Most people like order and feel empowered in organized environments, at home or work," explains Jan Cisek, environmental psychologist and feng shui expert (fengshuilondon.net). "Physical environments are relatively easy to control, and this gives people a sense of power." The need for clarity is a natural response to a confusing and often threatening world out there. Creating a bit of order in our homes and workplaces can give us a sense that it will all be all right in the end. "But decluttering can do more than help you feel in control; it can actually lower your levels of the stress hormone cortisol." Research shows that women living amid physical clutter not only have raised stress levels but are also more likely to feel depressed.

Those who described their homes as "restful" or "tidy" had lower cortisol levels, according to the UCLA study. The less clutter a person has, the higher their life satisfaction and sense of home, according to recent research published in the *Journal of Environmental Psychology*. Clutter is a visual distraction that competes for your attention, wearing down your ability to focus by limiting your brain's ability to process information. Spring-clean your surroundings and you'll feel mentally clearer and more decisive, the research suggests. And it's best to keep on top of your things before they mount up. "People become overwhelmed and can't then make decisions on what to keep or discard," explains study author and psychology professor Joseph Ferrari at DePaul University. This indecision often results in putting things off. Ferrari's latest research showed that people who procrastinate tend to live in cluttered surroundings.

Becoming clutter-free has another benefit too. Others see you as more capable, caring, and conscientious if you keep your surroundings tidy. A messy office tends to make people think you are uncaring and neurotic, according to new research from the University of Michigan. Clearing the decks can even help your diet. Those who work in a tidy space were twice as likely to choose an apple over a chocolate bar as those in a messy office, according to a study in the journal *Psychological Science*. But what if you actually thrive on disorganized chaos? The advice is: "Don't sweat it!". Minimalism isn't for everyone, and if you're comfortable in your clutter and it doesn't stress you, there is no reason to feel guilty or devote more time to tidying. Some research even suggests a bit of chaos can actually make you more creative. But if you're ready to do it, choose a method that inspires you. Whether it's the Kondo style, roping in a friend, or hiring a professional, the key is to make a start. Also, don't be hard on yourself if you feel overwhelmed. Celebrate whatever items you do manage to clear!

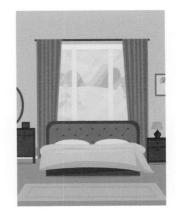

DON'T FORGET A DIGI-DECLUTTER

If you dread switching on your phone or laptop to an overload of emails, texts, tweets, posts or messages, here's what to do:

- Start with your social networking activities. Delete any dormant or irrelevant accounts you may have and minimize your friends, followers, and who you follow, making sure you only have relevant ones (or at least review your settings so you don't receive their updates).
- Spring-clean your emails by unsubscribing to newsletters that no longer interest you, and organize the rest of them into folders.

STEP ONE
Bedroom bliss

How you start your day matters. Just a few minutes spent clearing bedside clutter and planning what to wear the night before can create a calm morning and determine how you feel for the rest of the day. "Anything you can do to save headspace in the morning will help you feel energized and ready for the day," says professional declutterer Kate Ibbotson (atidymind.co.uk). Put clothes away or in the laundry and lay out your outfit for the next day—even down to your underwear. It will save precious minutes in the morning. Sleeping amid clutter isn't conducive to rest and relaxation, so aim to keep your bedside table and under the bed clear and tidy. "Tackle this by having a clear 'home' for everything," suggests Kate. "If you find that the same things tend to gather on your bedside table, then intentionally create a home for them. For example, have a special dish for loose earrings."

STEP TWO
Simply clean

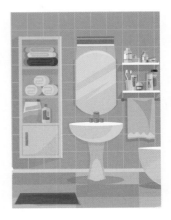

As the first room you enter in the morning and the last one you go to before bed, your bathroom can set the tone for the beginning and end of your day. Gather all your toiletries together and have a cull. "Keep only what you love, regularly use and that suits your skin and hair," says Kate. "And avoid bulk buying—the storage it takes up is rarely worth the money you've saved." Try keeping a streamlined make-up bag containing just the everyday essentials so you don't have to rummage through everything. And replace any scratchy or threadbare towels that have seen better days. "Don't underestimate the pleasure of a soft towel in the morning to add a little luxury to your day," says Kate.

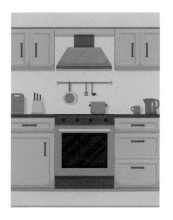

STEP THREE
Tidy kitchen

Clearing out cupboards and surfaces in your kitchen can save time in the mornings and will also help you make healthier food choices throughout the day. When both healthy and unhealthy options are available, people eat double the amount of unhealthy snacks when they're in a cluttered kitchen than in a tidy one, according to research published in the Journal of Environment and Behaviour. Start by clearing out the cupboards, ditching duplicate spices and jams, and letting go of items you don't use. Next, clear the work surfaces, keeping out only electrical items you use all the time such as the kettle and toaster. "Have a permanent home for your keys such as a hook or tray and a "catch-all" box or shelf for everyday essentials such as your wallet," suggests Kate. "Assign a home for every little thing to avoid your drawers becoming dumping grounds."

GO MINIMAL

Ask yourself: How might my life be better with less? By answering this question, you identify the benefits of letting go—not only how, but the more important why. Understanding the purpose of decluttering will grant you the leverage to keep going until you reach the freedom of having only what you need.

Start small. Once you understand why you're decluttering, get momentum by starting small. We recommend the 30-day minimalism game. Find a friend who's willing to play. Each person gets rid of one thing they do not need on the first day of the month, two on the second, three on the third, and so on. Every possession must be out of your house by midnight each day (or in the recycling or "take-to-the-thrift-store-when-I-can" piles). Whoever keeps it going the longest wins!

Reassess value. Ask yourself: how important is the stuff in my life? Take a moment and write down your 10 most expensive material possessions from the last decade—car, house, jewelry, furniture, and any other material things. Next to that list, make another top-10 list: things that add the most value to your life. Be honest with yourself when you're making these lists; it's likely that the two lists have nothing in common.

Enforce the 90/90 rule. Look at a possession—pick something; anything. Have you used that item in the last 90 days? If you haven't, will you use it in the next 90 days? If not, it's OK to let it go.

Organize. No matter where you are on your journey, remember that the easiest way to organize your stuff is to get rid of most of it. Imagine the space it will create, physical and mental.

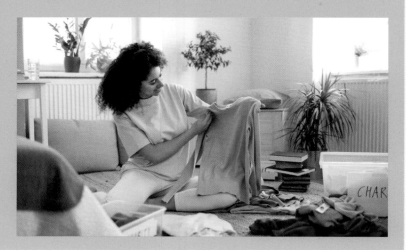

STEP FOUR
Calm commute

If you travel to your workplace, it pays to minimize the stress of clutter on your commute so that you get to work ready to have a great day. The best way to experience a clutter-free commute that will energize your day is to walk or cycle to work. Spending time outdoors in nature has been shown to boost your mood and immune system, and to lower stress levels. Multiple studies back this up. If you commute by car, keep it clean by getting into the habit of taking everything out of your vehicle at the end of each day and investing in a car bin or rubbish bag to keep litter in one place.

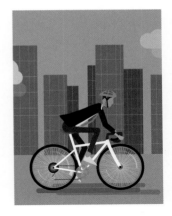

STEP FIVE
Work space serenity

Wherever you work, a clutter-free zone can boost productivity, help you focus, and prompt healthier habits. Studies have shown that when we are surrounded by clutter, we find it harder to read people's feelings and think clearly, and easier to give in to calorie-laden comfort food. Take half an hour to clear up your desk and you'll reap the wellbeing rewards. While you're at it, tweak your environment to favour healthy habits. Switch your screensaver to a photograph of nature; even pictures of green space activate the parasympathetic nervous system, thereby lowering stress, according to research from the Netherlands. If you work in a public space such as a school, shop, or hospital, simply having a micro-space that's all yours (even just a neat, tidy locker or corner of the staff room) can help you feel calmer and more in control.

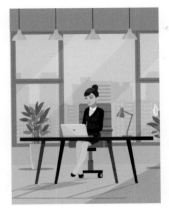

STEP SIX
Organized entrance

The quickest route to calm evenings is an organized entry. Find a spot for everything so that you're not battling through piles of shoes and coats just to get in! "If you have a hallway, create drop zones for shoes, coats and bags by attaching hooks to walls, fitting storage with cubby holes and high wall shelving for umbrellas, gloves, and hats," says Kate. "Then you can put your things in their places in a few small movements." The aim is to create a calm, clear entry point that won't make your stress hormones spike and will set you up for an easy-going evening.

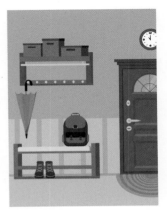

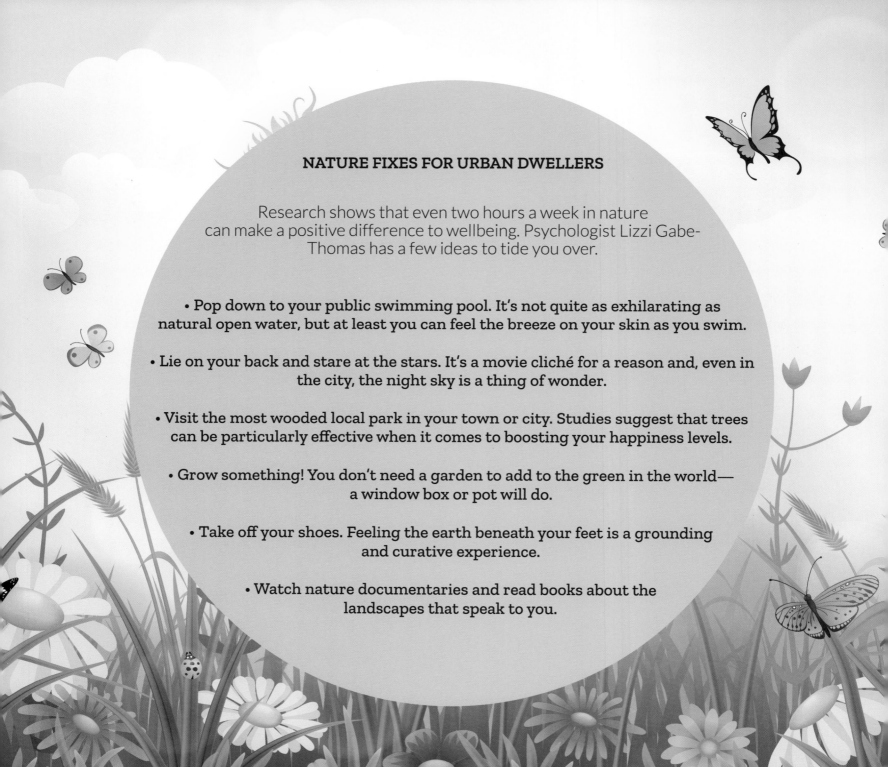

NATURE FIXES FOR URBAN DWELLERS

Research shows that even two hours a week in nature can make a positive difference to wellbeing. Psychologist Lizzi Gabe-Thomas has a few ideas to tide you over.

- Pop down to your public swimming pool. It's not quite as exhilarating as natural open water, but at least you can feel the breeze on your skin as you swim.

- Lie on your back and stare at the stars. It's a movie cliché for a reason and, even in the city, the night sky is a thing of wonder.

- Visit the most wooded local park in your town or city. Studies suggest that trees can be particularly effective when it comes to boosting your happiness levels.

- Grow something! You don't need a garden to add to the green in the world— a window box or pot will do.

- Take off your shoes. Feeling the earth beneath your feet is a grounding and curative experience.

- Watch nature documentaries and read books about the landscapes that speak to you.

SET A ROUTINE

With a few simple lifestyle tweaks, you can be firing on all cylinders from the moment you wake up until the end of the day! Here's one possible routine.

🕕 6.00 am BE PREDICTABLE

The most effective way to stamp out sluggishness is also the simplest—get up at the same time every day. While this may be bad news for lovers of the weekend lie-in, experts agree that if you can be consistent with wake-up times seven days a week, you'll rise feeling more rested. Boost your ability to bounce out of bed by opening the curtains and getting natural light as soon as you can. This will help your body know it's time to wake up.

Below: A bowl of oatmeal topped with fruits of the forest will set you up for the day ahead. It is a healthy breakfast option that releases its energy slowly, keeping you fuller for longer.

🕖 7.00 am MOVE YOUR BODY

There are some serious perks to adopting a morning exercise habit. Research shows that morning workouts can raise cortisol, boosting focus, mental clarity and energy levels for hours afterwards. Early exercise will also lift your mood, even if you're reluctant to get moving. Furthermore, a morning sweat session can have a knock-on effect on the rest of your day, making you generally more active and less likely to experience food cravings, according to research at Brigham Young University.

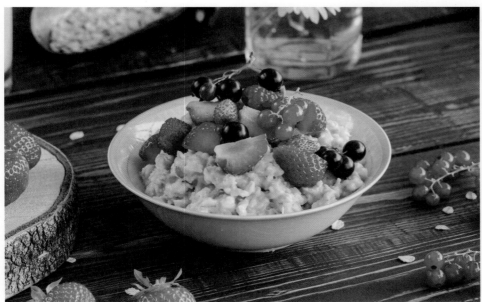

🕗 8.00 am BE BRILLIANT AT BREAKFAST

Make the most of your revved up post-workout metabolism by eating a nutritious breakfast to restore glucose levels and give your brain fuel to focus. "Aim for around 400 calories for breakfast, which is about 20 percent of daily energy requirements," advises Emily Robinson, nutrition scientist at the British Nutrition Foundation. "Include higher-fiber, wholegrain starchy carbohydrates such as oats." Also, try to eat some fruit or veg and a source of protein such as nuts, eggs or beans to help to keep you going through the morning. Avoid sugary cereals and processed foods, which will only make you feel sluggish.

🕐 10.30 am TIME YOUR CAFFEINE INTAKE

If you time your coffee break to work with your body's cortisol levels, you'll get a bigger energy boost, according to neuroscientists at Harvard. Have coffee or tea between 9.30am and 11.30am when your levels of cortisol—the hormone that helps to regulate metabolism—are at their highest. If caffeine no longer gives you an energy jolt, you may be building up a tolerance, so swap your coffee for a hike up and down the stairs. Ten minutes of stair-climbing will make you feel more energetic than a coffee break, according to research from the University of Georgia.

🕐 1.00 pm GET OUTSIDE

You're halfway through your day and now's the time to reclaim your lunch break and go outdoors. Even the smallest nugget of nature can unleash serious benefits on those who make time for it. Being in a green space has been shown to lower stress levels and boost memory and concentration. In a study at the University of Michigan, students performed better in memory and attention tests after a walk in a park, compared to those who strolled city streets. If you must eat "al desko," at least switch your screen saver to an inspiring natural view or have a plant nearby, as recent research indicates that even seeing pictures of nature can increase your energy levels.

Below: Cold water has been found to increase the production of mood-elevating hormones and neurotransmitters that can improve symptoms of depression and anxiety. If you can't face total immersion in an outdoor swimming pool or the sea, splashing cold water on your wrists or face also does the trick.

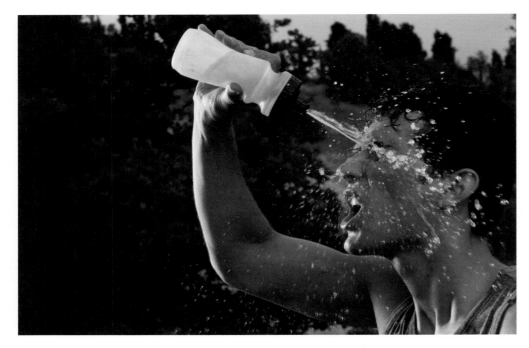

🕐 3.00 pm BRAVE THE COLD!

The evidence for cold water therapies to fight fatigue just keeps on coming. Cold water has been shown to boost alertness and may even combat depression and long-term exhaustion. Although much of the research has centred on endorphin-releasing icy blasts in the shower, you can get a mini energy jolt by splashing cold water on your wrists or face, where you have a high concentration of nerve endings. While you're at it, top up your water bottle. Staying hydrated is essential to feeling energized, and not drinking enough during the day may even disrupt sleep. New research suggests those who get six hours or fewer a night could be dehydrated. Aim for 1–2 liters a day. Keep forgetting? Stay on track with a free reminder app such as Daily Water.

🕐 5.00 pm FOCUS ON WHAT YOU'VE FINISHED

Fretting over unfinished tasks or how much you still have to do is a major energy drainer, so take five minutes at the end of the working day to flip that focus and appreciate what you have achieved. "The feeling of having too many tabs open in your brain is a sure-fire way to exhaustion," says Dr. Libby Weaver, author of Exhausted to Energized. Instead, notice what went well today and what you did achieve, however small.

🕕 6.00 pm PLUG INTO YOUR PLAYLIST

Fading fast? Plug yourself into a high-energy playlist. Research suggests that music has a direct effect on your body by stimulating the autonomic nervous system, which controls breathing, heartbeat, and digestive processes. It can also light up the feel-good networks in your brain. "We know that music activates reward and pleasure networks in the brain, including dopamine levels, which impact emotion and short-term mood," explains David Greenberg, a psychologist at Cambridge University.

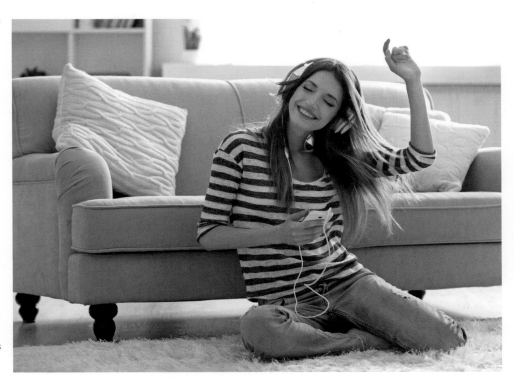

Above: Listening to music is a great way to improve your mood immediately. Your favorite songs or pieces of music can evoke memories, reduce stress and help you to express yourself.

🕖 7.00 pm BE SOCIAL YET SPONTANEOUS!

Skip the sofa and get socializing. After work is the time to go for a walk with a friend, join a club, or volunteer; being social helps you bounce off the energy of others. Maximize your enjoyment by keeping it somewhat spontaneous.

🕙 10.00 pm MAKE TIME TO MEDITATE

For an energized day it helps to prepare a little the night before. So, before bed, opt for a spot of meditation or breathwork, as both can calm your mind and help you drift off to sleep. Just 25 minutes of yoga or meditation is enough to see these benefits, according to research from the University of Waterloo in Canada. By focusing your brain's conscious processing power on the breath, your mind blocks out the noise of non-essential thoughts. Chances are you'll nod off before you know it!

AND BREATHE

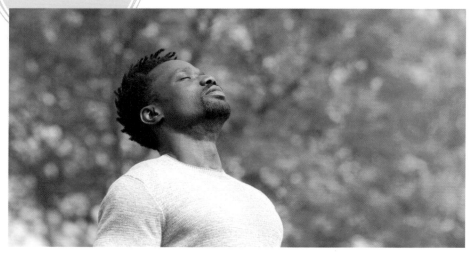

Breathing is so automatic that you tend not to think about how it affects your body. But read on to discover how breathing better could be the key to transforming your life.

You take around 20,000 breaths a day. Considering how vital it is, it's a simple process. Breathing in makes your diaphragm tighten and move down, making space for your lungs to take in air. Oxygen from this air passes through your lungs into your blood vessels to circulate through your body. At the same time, carbon dioxide moves from the bloodstream into your lungs. On your exhale, the diaphragm goes back upwards, pushing that carbon dioxide out and into the air. Ideally, you should fill your lungs with as much air as you can—that's 3-4 liters (5–7 pints)!—pulling the air down deep into your lungs. Then you should exhale fully so the used-up gases leave your lungs, creating maximum room for another oxygen-filled breath.

The problem is many of us aren't doing this effectively. Most people breathe in only around 500ml of air per breath. "About 90–95 percent of people don't use their lower muscles to breathe, instead only using the secondary muscles in the upper part of the chest that should normally only kick in when you need to breathe quickly," explains breath expert Richie Bostock, aka The Breath Guy (thebreathguy.co.uk). Chances are you rarely exhale fully, so you never completely exchange all the used gas for fresh new air that powers your body.

A PHYSICAL BOOST

How exactly can breathing well benefit you? Let's start with the physical changes. "The movement of your diaphragm acts as an internal massage to your body's organs—this helps stimulate the natural removal of toxic by-products," says Claire Dale, co-author of Physical Intelligence. Breathing well has also been proven to positively affect immunity. At least two studies have shown that slow, controlled breathing directly triggers a release of anti-inflammatory compounds by your immune system.

ALTER YOUR BODY
"What people don't realize is that correct breathing is the most underrated way to shift the way you think and feel," says Richie. "When you breathe effectively, you create changes in your nervous system and an exchange of gases in your blood that can directly alter your body both physically and mentally."

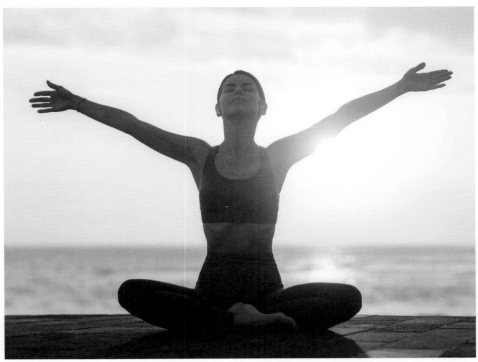

Breathing efficiently also floods your body with the oxygen it needs to thrive, while preventing a build-up of carbon dioxide that can leave you sluggish. "If you want to energize your system, one of the easiest ways to do it is with the breath," says Claire. "Correct breathing can also improve how you think. Teaching people to breathe in a steady manner actually led to a 62 percent increase in cognitive capacity and complex reasoning in one South African study. "Not only is increased oxygen a likely reason for this, but effective breathing actually changed the patterns of brain waves, producing fewer waves associated with scattered thinking and more waves that led to focus." Good breathing also calms your body. When you're stressed you hold your breath and breathe in a shallow manner. "This leads to a build-up of carbon dioxide, which then raises cortisol levels, increasing your anxiety," says Claire. "Slowing and deepening your breathing is therefore one of the easiest ways to reduce stress." It also has a knock-on effect of lowering blood pressure.

Above: *See if you can find an outdoor space to practice your breathing. The feel of the sun on your skin and the wind on your face will help you to connect with nature, leading to an amazing array of effects: more energy, a happier mood, reduced stress, enhanced attention, improved immunity, and a better quality of sleep.*

THE MENTAL BENEFITS

Every emotion has a precise breathing pattern. "When we're angry, we huff and puff; when we sob, we expel air in tiny bursts, then take a huge gulp of air inwards; laughter is just quick, rapid breathing," says Richie. The link between breath pattern and emotional state is so strong that in one study at Belgium's University of Louvain, people asked to breathe in a "happy" or "angry" way ended up feeling that way simply because they'd changed their breath pattern. The direct ability for your breath to change how you feel has led to the development of breathwork—techniques where the breath pattern is manipulated to help change emotional states. "You can use the breath to generate feelings you may have suppressed and then release them. This can literally change people's lives," says Richie. It's often the way that the most seemingly simple things, such as breathing, can have the most profound impact. But to see benefits you have to remember to make changes and do it consistently. By making a more conscious effort to tune in to how you are breathing—perhaps by setting an alarm on your phone every hour or half hour—you could begin to transform the way you feel in both body and mind, and it won't cost you a penny.

Below: Breathwork is simple yet powerful, and it's a good idea to teach children how to do it. Once they have the tools for slowing their breathing and heart rate, they'll instantly feel calmer and will be better equipped to deal with big emotions such as anger, frustration, and disappointment.

It can help to consider the following when thinking about your breathing:

SPEED: "The speed at which you breathe directly influences your nervous system," says Claire. "Slowing your breathing will calm you down. If you wish to energize yourself, you can breathe a little faster. Normal breathing has a pace of about 12–14 breaths per minute; to calm your body drop down to 5–7 per minute; to energize, speed it up to 15–16."

DEPTH: This is the vital part of good breathwork. "You need to breathe deep into your lungs, so your diaphragm moves up and down," explains Claire. Try to expand your belly and ribs as you inhale and press them back in as you exhale.

MOUTH OR NOSE: "Mouth breathers get a bad rap," says Claire. Inhaling through your mouth is the best way to get a lot of air into your lungs quickly, but it's better to inhale through your nose as this stimulates your calming parasympathetic system. It also warms the air and filters out some pollutants and germs.

IN/OUT RATIO: For normal breathing, your exhale should be slightly longer than your inhale. A count of four seconds in and seven seconds out is ideal.

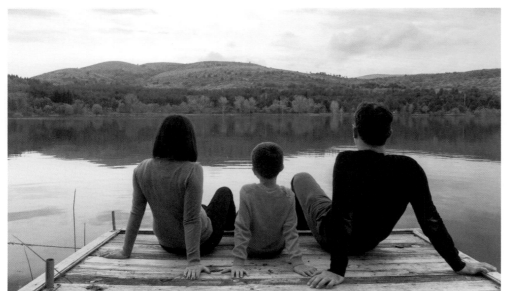

BREATHWORK TECHNIQUES

Breathwork is the catch-all name for using the breath to directly change your body in some way. Here are three techniques to try.

PACED BREATHING: This is a slow, steady, regular type of breathing for tackling stress, anxiety, hot flushes and insomnia. It helps promote calm and re-educates your body on the correct way to breathe. Inhale and exhale slowly and steadily 5–7 times a minute. Practice for 10 minutes, twice a day.

PRANAYAMA: This is the word used for the different types of breathwork used in yoga practice—it might include the rapid, energizing rhythm of bellows breath or the more calming, alternate nostril breathing. Sit on a chair and block your right nostril with your right thumb, inhale through the left and then in a smooth movement, block the left nostril with your ring finger while releasing the right nostril and breathing out through that side. Then inhale slowly through the right and repeat the process. Keep going for 3–5 minutes. This type of breathing directly activates the parasympathetic nervous system, calming your body.

MINDFUL BREATHING: This is the practice of focusing on your breath as a form of meditation. You don't control it, you simply notice it and sometimes count it. Focus on the sound of your breath, the rise and fall of your chest and the temperature of the air as it enters your nostrils. After the first exhale, silently count "one", then on the next exhale count "two" all the way up to 10. Then begin at one again. It sounds easy but it's difficult to reach 10 without your mind wandering!

TIGHTEN YOUR BOUNDARIES

Boundaries are important because they keep us safe—just like fences around our houses.

Having clear boundaries demonstrates that we have self-respect and limits about what we are prepared to accept and do. It might be helpful to ask a few close friends to look at the list below and give you feedback about how many of these habits you exhibit:

- You apologize a lot.
- You agree to things that make you uncomfortable or that you don't want to do.
- You put others' needs before your own.
- You resent that you're being taken advantage of.
- You allow people to take advantage of you.
- You have difficulty saying no.
- You fall on your sword to avoid upsetting others.
- You fear conflict and avoid difficult conversations.

Complete the following sentences and keep your list of boundaries with you so you can read it regularly and learn to exercise them:

- I have the right to...
- I will not accept...
- I will not choose to spend time with people who...
  - If I'm asked to do something I don't want to do, I will...
    - I will not continue relationships with people who...
    - Having clear boundaries will enable me to...

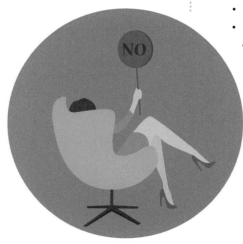

PREPARE FOR ACTION

If you are not used to asserting yourself, you might want to practice it a few times before you do it for real. Ask two friends to help you have a dress rehearsal—make it fun and playful! One can play the part of the person you are going to be speaking to, and the other can play the role of observer. The observer can stop you to tell you to change your posture or the inflection in your voice, so you look and sound stronger.

MIX THINGS UP!

If you ever feel bored or in a rut, making even small changes to your daily routine can really help to mix things up.

Change is a constant in life and there are always going to be factors outside of our control: world events, other people, the weather. Learning to flex and adapt to changing circumstances takes time and practice, but equips us for life and its uncertainties. Trying to control everything will not stop unexpected things from happening; it will only make you more anxious. To become more bendy willow tree than rigid oak, start small and be kind to yourself with the following approaches:

- Do a new form of exercise.
- Get dressed in a different order.
- Cook a new recipe.
- Question the way you have always done things and make small changes to your usual pattern of behavior. Get curious about the outcome.

RELEASE YOUR INNER CHILD

If you find that your life is all work and no play, think about getting in touch with your inner child for a day. Laughing, playing and spending time doing things just for pleasure can reduce your stress levels.

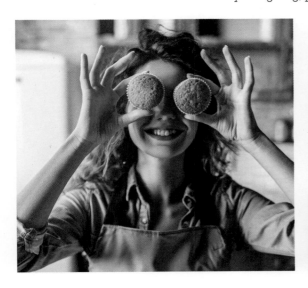

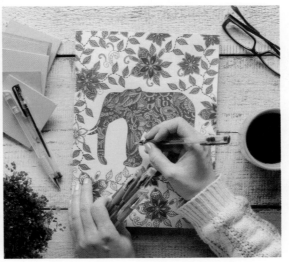

Children are in touch with their feelings and needs, moment by moment. Releasing your inner child can put you back in touch with what you really want, so you can have a break from thinking about others' needs. Ask yourself: "What would I like to eat today?" Forget about social convention—anything goes! Go for a walk with no destination. Drift around, look up and notice things you've not noticed before. Watch a children's film or a cartoon. Do some coloring in—outside the lines if you want!

STRESS-BUSTING SOLUTIONS

There are plenty of ways you can knock stress on the head. Here are a few ideas to try—and you'll find plenty more in the next chapter too!

PAT A PUPPY, CUDDLE A KITTEN

A pet is for life, not just for Christmas, but if you ever happen to acquire a new cat or dog, it's great news for your stress levels! Playing with an animal not only gets you moving around, but petting one has also been shown to reduce levels of cortisol by a study at the University of Missouri Columbia. If you love dogs but don't have one yourself, Borrow my Doggy (borrowmydoggy.com) can connect you with local dog owners who need help with walks and dog-sitting. Or just simply go for a walk in your local park and admire all the carefree canines enjoying their walks.

SNIFF A LOVELY SCENT

Next time you're borrowing your other half's snuggly jumper, tell yourself it's all part of a stress-busting plan. Smelling a romantic partner's scent is proven to help lower stress levels, according to researchers at the University of British Columbia. If you don't have a partner (or just don't fancy sniffing their dirty laundry!), the fragrances of lavender, jasmine, and green apple are all also said to help alleviate stress—and might be slightly more pleasant! It might be time to get out that scented candle you received in your stocking last Christmas.

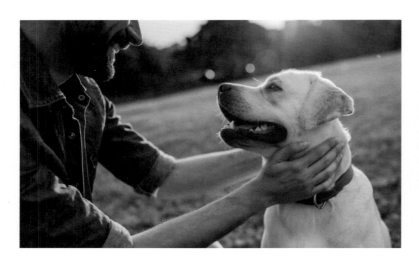
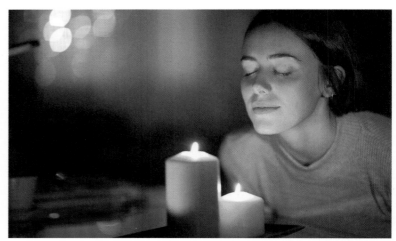

BLOW UP A BALLOON

We associate balloons with happy memories, but they can also help us stay relaxed and healthy every day. By using a balloon and slowly inflating it and deflating it, you will naturally force yourself to start taking deep, soothing breaths. Your body needs oxygen to feel calm, but when you're worrying, you tend to take quick, shallow breaths, So this technique is really helpful.

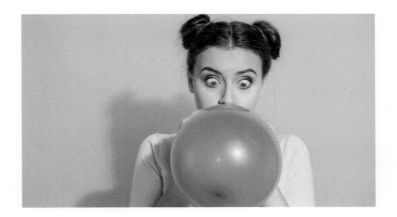

SCHEDULE YOUR STRESS

It might sound counterintuitive, but scheduling a specific "worry session" into your day could reduce your overall stress levels, according to a study published in the Journal of Psychotherapy and Psychosomatics. Using a diary planner to organize and structure your days should help you to feel less rushed and flustered, but if you still feel panic rising, allot your worries to a specific half-hour window. This should help you feel as if you're controlling your stress, instead of it controlling you.

TUNE INTO NATURE

Getting out into the fresh air, surrounded by nature, is a brilliant mood booster and stress reliever. But even just watching wildlife videos will help you harness similar mental health benefits, according to a study by the University of California. There are wildlife webcams all over the world that you can access online. Why not pay a visit to a wildlife website where you can see live footage of garden wildlife, birds of prey, native mammals, and much more?

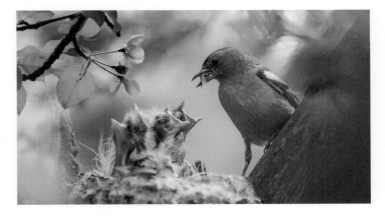

JOIN A CHOIR

Choirs are soaring in popularity at the moment, and no wonder—they're fun, sociable, and might just be your ultimate stress buster. Singing with others triggers the release of oxytocin, a "happy hormone" that helps lower stress levels and blood pressure, according to Swedish research. Popchoir (popchoir.com) holds community choirs, where you'll find yourself belting out anything from Lady Gaga to Coldplay. There's no audition process, so every voice is welcome.

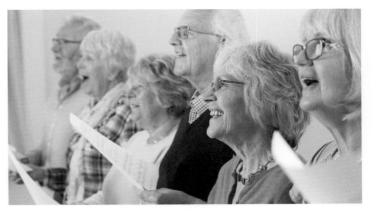

FRIENDS FOREVER

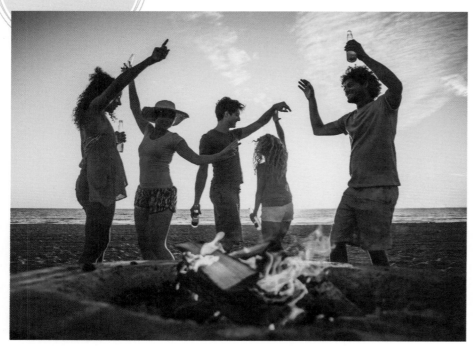

Good chums warm your heart—and they can make it healthier too!

A SOCIAL NETWORK

The scientific evidence is mounting for the idea that friends are good for our hearts and our long-term health. In fact, loneliness and social isolation have been shown to increase your risk of a heart attack by 29 percent and your chance of a stroke by 32 percent—so a lack of friends is just as dangerous for your heart as smoking or obesity. When life gets hectic it's easy for friendships to take a back seat, but today's busy lifestyles are all the more reason for us to make the effort to see our close friends. On average we have fewer friends now than our parents' generation did, despite having many more ways to connect, according to research from Cornell University in the US. And this could be to the detriment of our health and wellbeing. "Social support has a positive effect on our heart health and our health in general," says health psychologist Dr. Megan Arroll (drmegarroll.com). "Friends can help you stay healthy in practical ways by encouraging you to eat better, being your gym buddy, and helping you through stressful times, but it also goes deeper than that." The perception of a good social network is incredibly important. Feeling loved and cared for, having people to rely on and knowing you have this back-up is as, if not more, important than the practical help your friends give you.

THE FRIENDS EFFECT

When you spend time with friends who make you happy, many of your body's systems undergo positive changes. "People with good support systems and friendships have lower levels of urinary catecholamines, which are hormones made by your adrenal glands that are released into your blood stream when you're physically or emotionally stressed," says Dr. Arroll. "They make you breathe faster, raise your blood pressure, and send more blood to major organs, including your brain, heart, and kidneys. Having friends to turn to during difficult times could buffer the damaging effects of stress on your body," says Dr. Sheldon Cohen, a psychologist at Carnegie Mellon University who has been exploring the links between relationships and health for more than three decades. That chat on the phone, or a quick coffee with a friend helps lower your cortisol level, which has a positive knock-on effect on your immune and neuroendocrine systems. "Although cortisol is an important part of your stress response (which we need for survival), your levels should dip over a 24-hour period so that you can switch off, relax and sleep soundly," says Dr. Arroll. "Knowing you have the support of your social network raises your oxytocin levels to decrease the amount of cortisol rushing around your body, lowering blood pressure and switching on the parasympathetic nervous system, which dampens the stress response so that your body can relax even more." What more excuse do you need for a fun night out?

I'LL BE THERE FOR YOU

You could argue that we're better connected with our friends and families now than we've ever been before. After all, social media allows us to keep in touch with loved ones all across the world. But these online connections aren't all necessarily beneficial. On average we have 155 friends on Facebook, but in a crisis we feel we could turn to just four people for help, according to research by Oxford University. "Genuine friends are very important, and nothing compares to proper face-to-face contact," says Dr. Arroll. "Social media has quite a bad reputation at the moment in terms of its impact on mental health, but research shows that if you use it to really connect with people, rather than just passively scrolling and liking posts, it can be a good way to maintain friendships." "Keep in mind that how your peers present themselves on social media might not be a true reflection of their lives," says Dr. Cohen. "People often present an exaggerated and positive version of their world—a happy marriage, successful job, perfect families, which can result in you making destructive comparisons." This could increase your stress levels and have a negative impact on your health and wellbeing, whereas when you meet a friend in "real life" you're much more likely to get the unedited version of events and benefit from shared experiences. "The real health benefits come from close friends and confidants, which your average friend on social media generally isn't," says Dr. Cohen.

PHONE A FRIEND

Making the effort to stay in touch with your friends and going out and meeting new people really is worth it. "If you have a very busy schedule and it's not practical to meet face-to-face, speaking on the phone is one way to make that human connection," says Arroll. "Speaking on the phone allows you to hear the tone, intonation and volume of a friend's voice—all of which give us important cues to how someone is truly feeling and thinking, so we feel supported and loved." This isn't possible online, even with a million emojis! "Make the most of opportunities to make

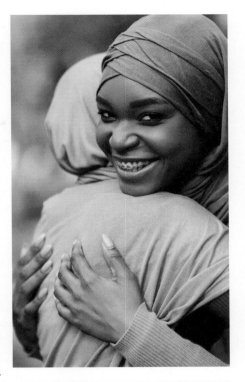

HUG IT OUT
Give your friends a hug when you see them for even more health benefits. A cuddle could help to lower blood pressure, reduce stress levels and cause the release of happy hormone oxytocin to boost your mood and feelings of wellbeing. Hang on for a little longer than average, though—it takes at least 20 seconds for those blood pressure benefits to kick in.

new friends when they come your way too—it really is a case of 'the more the merrier.'" We've found that the more diverse people's social networks are—the more types of connections they had—the less likely they were to develop a cold after exposure to a virus," says Dr. Cohen. People with plenty of friends tend to look after their health better, avoiding things like smoking and drinking, and instead having a more positive outlook. "It's a good ideate try to belong to different groups, to volunteer in different ways and be involved in your neighborhood if you can," says Dr. Cohen. "Involvement with other people across diverse situations can have a very potent, very positive effect on your health."

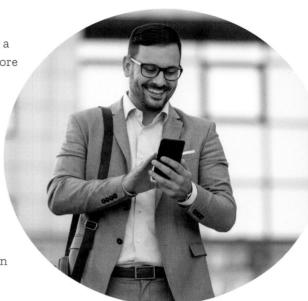

THE FIVE PHASES OF FRIENDSHIP

Relationship experts have identified a chronological pattern to bonding and establishing an enduring and valuable friendship:

- Curiosity. You know the drill. You meet someone in a social situation and something about them gets your attention. You want to get to know them better.
- Exploration. This happens as you spend time together expanding on that initial attraction. This phase can feel like dating—a flurry of excited texts and a buzz when you think about being in each other's company, unpicking your shared values and interests.
- Familiarity develops when there's an understanding between fledgling friends—you are doing activities together and hanging out, simply enjoying each other's company.
- Vulnerability comes from trust. The more comfortable we feel with another person, the more likely we are to show the sides of ourselves we might usually reserve for loved ones.
- Intimacy is the fifth stage of friendship—the end goal, if you like. It tends to happen when there's been vulnerability on both sides. Intimacy comes from a place of implicit trust, but usually takes time, so be patient.

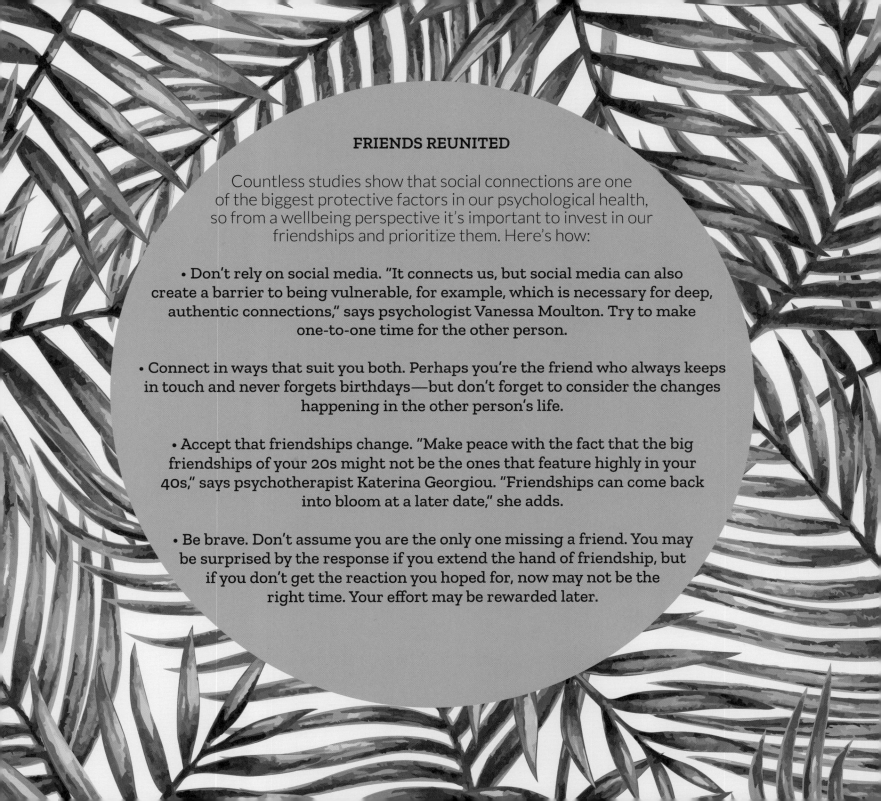

FRIENDS REUNITED

Countless studies show that social connections are one
of the biggest protective factors in our psychological health,
so from a wellbeing perspective it's important to invest in our
friendships and prioritize them. Here's how:

• Don't rely on social media. "It connects us, but social media can also
create a barrier to being vulnerable, for example, which is necessary for deep,
authentic connections," says psychologist Vanessa Moulton. Try to make
one-to-one time for the other person.

• Connect in ways that suit you both. Perhaps you're the friend who always keeps
in touch and never forgets birthdays—but don't forget to consider the changes
happening in the other person's life.

• Accept that friendships change. "Make peace with the fact that the big
friendships of your 20s might not be the ones that feature highly in your
40s," says psychotherapist Katerina Georgiou. "Friendships can come back
into bloom at a later date," she adds.

• Be brave. Don't assume you are the only one missing a friend. You may
be surprised by the response if you extend the hand of friendship, but
if you don't get the reaction you hoped for, now may not be the
right time. Your effort may be rewarded later.

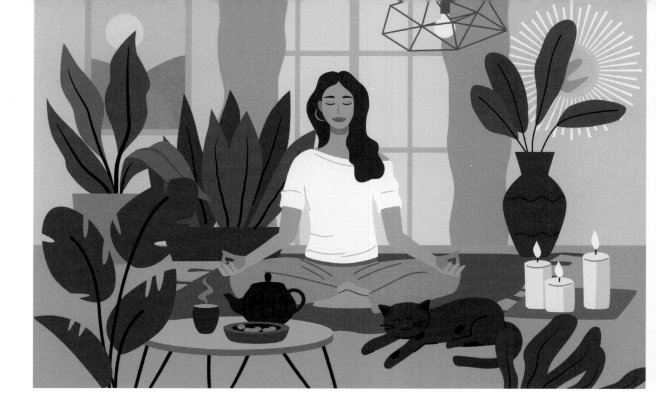

MOVE ON WITH A HOPEFUL HEART

Had your heart broken? Try our tips from Relate counsellor Simone Bose to find positivity and optimism, even after a difficult break-up.

1. **Allow yourself time.** There will always be sadness and hurt when a relationship ends, and those feelings need to be processed. Don't expect to give or receive a glowing review of your ex immediately. Give it time.
2. **Write things down.** Make a list of all the things that were positive about the relationship, so they don't drown in a sea of negatives. The act of writing things down also reinforces more positive thinking.
3. **Create a timeline.** This allows you to see your relationship as a whole and recognize that there were good times at various stages along the way. Don't focus all your attention on the end of the relationship as it started to break down.

4. **Identify the benefits.** Whether it's children, friends, security or personal growth, most relationships give you something. Think about what you have gained and what your partner has gained from you.
5. **See opportunity as well as loss.** Your future may not be panning out as you imagined it would just yet, but it's still your future. Hold onto what you got out of the relationship and use it to create a new life for yourself.

Self-love exercises
Simple ways to show yourself TLC as a single person:

- Write down the qualities you admire in other people, then find examples of times you've demonstrated these qualities.
- Plan a date night for yourself.
- Take yourself out to dinner, buy yourself flowers. Whatever you would like someone else to do, do it!
- Think back to what you loved to do as six-year-old, take yourself on an adventure and do it. Set an intention for what you want from your next relationship, write it down, and repeat it to yourself every morning.
- Spend time appreciating your body. Look in the mirror and find things you love about your physical being, your abilities, and strength.

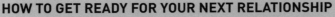

HOW TO GET READY FOR YOUR NEXT RELATIONSHIP
- Make a list of things that annoy you in a relationship, then ask yourself why they irritate you.
- As yourself what need you have that isn't being met.
- Identify the role you tend to fulfil in a relationship (protector, homemaker or even drama creator—be honest!), then pick another role to explore in your next relationship.
- Consider a relationship that ended and write down the facts about why it ended. Note any stories that you're making up about it.
- Set an intention for your new partner. How do you want to feel in their presence? What will your relationship be like? When will it happen?
- Treat yourself as you expect others to treat you.

HOW TO CREATE A CAREER TIMELINE

The following exercise can help you prepare for an interview, write your resumé, build confidence during a career transition and plan a future career path. Ask someone you trust to do it with you.

This exercise works so much better than writing down the jobs you have done and trying to pull out your strengths and key achievements. It brings your career to life by literally walking through it.

- Dot five or six pieces of colored paper card like stepping stones around a room. If the weather is nice, do it outside. Now, stand on the stepping stone that represents your most recent job.
- Ask your friend to have pen and paper and to ask you to talk about your successes, skills, high points, positive qualities, things you learned, training you did, experiences you had and good feedback you received. Stand near the stepping stone and tell your story. Your friend should write down what you say on the stone.
- Do the same for each stepping stone until you're back at your first job—maybe a Saturday job you did while you were at university. Everything counts.
- Walk back to the present-day stone, gathering up all the realizations about your career, all you have achieved and how much you have to offer.

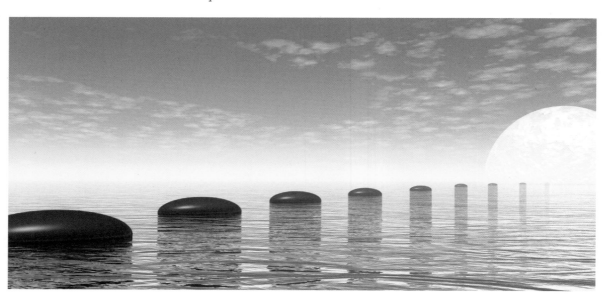

USE YOUR HUMAN RESOURCES

One of the bravest things we can do is to ask for help when in need. Think about people in your life who:

- Are great networkers and can connect you with others.
- Have information that may help you achieve your goal.
- Have experienced what you are going through.
- Will give you a loving kick up the backside if you need it.
- See the best in you and boost your confidence.

HOW TO FIND A FULFILLING ROLE:
PLEASURE, MEANING AND STRENGTHS

Here is a useful exercise to find out what you enjoy, what activities have meaning for you and what you're best at.

• Draw three large overlapping circles on a big piece of paper. Use three different-colored pens. Write one of these questions in each circle:

1. What gives me pleasure?

2. What gives me meaning?

3. What are my strengths?

• Put as many answers to these questions as you can in each of the circles. You don't have to do this in one sitting.

It is interesting to see the things that overlap in all three areas. You may want to use these as a checklist for when you're considering applying for jobs or changing career.

HOW TO FIND A JOB YOU LOVE

Want to transition to a career that fulfills you? Answer these "BRIDGE" questions first, says author Samantha Clarke.

Belief
In which area do you have little faith in your current job—the product, service, leadership style or company culture? Why?

Results
What does success look like to you? Do you want your boss's job? Are you motivated by rewards or recognition? Can you achieve what you want where you are?

Impact
What valuable knowledge or insight do you want to share? What's the biggest impact you would like to make? What would you like to be your legacy? Can you achieve it in the sector you are in?

Desire
In your present role, what do you want more of? Money, respect, status, stability, work that makes your heart sing or work/life harmony?

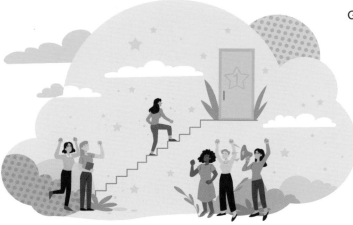

Growth
Is your industry burgeoning or shrinking? What are your prospects for finding a new job in a similar role? Is the company you work for in a tricky financial position?

Enrichment
How does your day-to-day experience make you feel? Do you feel competent, happy and enriched or unsuccessful, exhausted, bored, and restless? What are you absorbing and learning in your place of work at the moment?

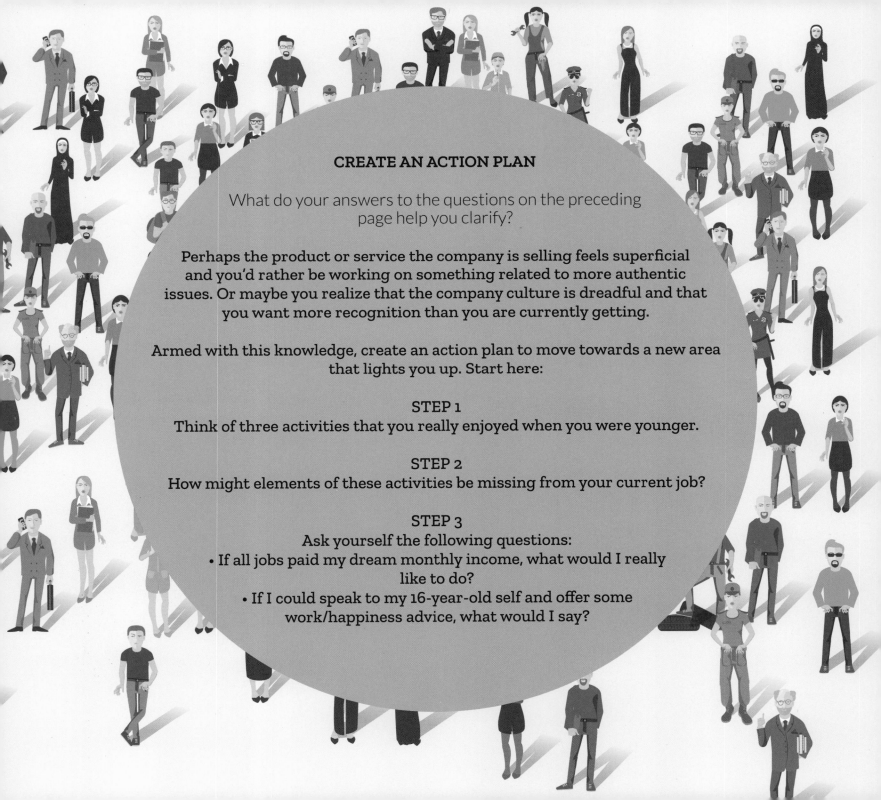

CREATE AN ACTION PLAN

What do your answers to the questions on the preceding page help you clarify?

Perhaps the product or service the company is selling feels superficial and you'd rather be working on something related to more authentic issues. Or maybe you realize that the company culture is dreadful and that you want more recognition than you are currently getting.

Armed with this knowledge, create an action plan to move towards a new area that lights you up. Start here:

STEP 1
Think of three activities that you really enjoyed when you were younger.

STEP 2
How might elements of these activities be missing from your current job?

STEP 3
Ask yourself the following questions:
• If all jobs paid my dream monthly income, what would I really like to do?
• If I could speak to my 16-year-old self and offer some work/happiness advice, what would I say?

THE MEANING OF SUCCESS

How do you get the life you want? A good place to start is to find out what success means to you. It's different for everyone!

Often, without realizing it, we strive for what is considered to be the standard version of success: family, kids, a good job, lots of money and a large house. In reality, we all have our own idea of what success should look and feel like, and for many of us it's not necessarily about material things. Of course, most of us like to have nice things, but success isn't solely about having a big house, a flashy car, and lots of money. You can have all of those things and still be miserable if you're in an unhappy relationship or you hate the job that enabled you to acquire them in the first place.

If you're not rich at the moment, you might think that money would make you happy. But there are downsides to having money. When you are rich, who can you trust? Are friends your friends because of your money? How do you keep your money? How do you keep making more of it to maintain your lifestyle? You may have had to work long, unsociable hours to get that money in the first place, and had to give up precious time with family and friends. You may have missed family birthdays and other important social occasions in the pursuit of success. And you may also feel the pressure to maintain your success and keep earning more money, so that you are perceived to be continually successful.

MONEY, MONEY, MONEY!
We don't need to conform to what society's definition of what being successful is. Success can't always be measured by money. In fact, if you talk to some of the world's richest people, they will often tell you that money hasn't made them happy.

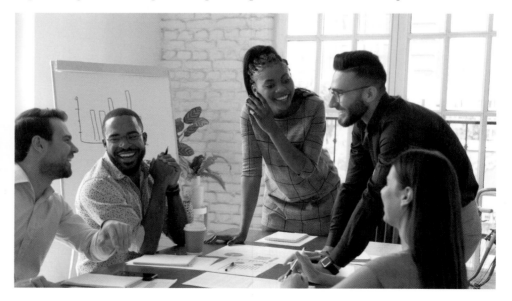

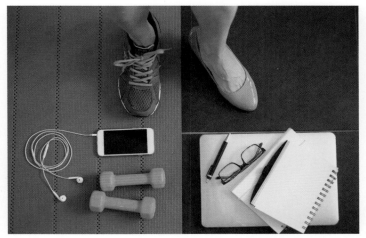

Money can also take its toll on your health. Sure, you might be able to afford good healthcare, but the price of getting rich for those who aren't fortunate enough to inherit money is hard work—long hours, in some cases, bad diet, no exercise, and relying on unhealthy vices like smoking and excessive drinking to unwind at the end of another ridiculously long day. Ask yourself, is this the kind of life you want for yourself? Is this really what success being about? And, of course, there are examples of very rich people who have died young, who would have traded every penny of their wealth to stay healthy. After all, money may be able to buy the best healthcare, but there are no guarantees when it comes to good health and wellbeing.

WORK/LIFE BALANCE

In order to get the life you want, the life that will make you feel happy, youthful and vibrant, you need to work out what success means to you. For some, it may mean working part-time and having spare time to spend with their family. For others, it could mean throwing themselves into a job or a career they absolutely love. For some people, it could mean having the time and freedom to travel and explore the world. Others may define success by having less money but more freedom to do the things they want to do.

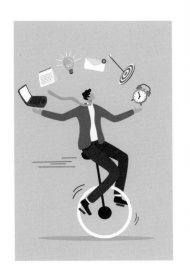

WHAT DO YOU WANT YOUR LIFE TO LOOK LIKE?

Here are some questions to consider when thinking about what success means to you and your work/life balance:

- What are you lacking in your life at the moment? Is it more time to spend with loved ones, a fresh challenge, or new purpose, or the opportunity to do a job that you enjoy?
- What activities do you most enjoy doing? When are you at your most relaxed and content?
- What sort of lifestyle would make you happy? Do you like the idea of a career in an area of business that you love, or would you rather have more downtime? Or would you like to have more time to improve your health and fitness?
- Is your current job fulfilling you? If not, what sort of job would you find rewarding? Write down three things that are most important to you. Also, think about what you haven't done yet.
- If you were to be told you only had a year to live, what things would be on your bucket list?

Once you have answered these questions, start working out how you can have more of these things in your life.

BECOME AN EXPERT NEGOTIATOR AT WORK

Want to get what you want in the workplace? Here's the lowdown on ways to get the deal of the decade!

• Find your zone of fairness. Pinpoint the overlap of what you need and what the other party is hoping for. The skill is recognizing the middle ground and agreeing on how to get there.

• Make your own needs clear and, at the same time, put yourself in the other person's shoes to understand the pressures on them. Get used to stating your position precisely, saying, for example: "I need a 20 percent reduction in fees to be able to continue using your service." Or "I'm looking for a time frame of less than three months to close this deal or I'll have to walk away."

• Be ready to walk away. When you're caught up in a negotiation, it can be hard to keep sight of the point at which an agreement is unacceptable, for example, when a price offer is too low. It is tough to reach this point and say no, simply because you've probably invested so much to get there, and it might be impossible to imagine not agreeing a deal. At these moments, step back, pause and seek advice. Find a mentor with whom to discuss it. The hardest part of negotiation is knowing when to walk away.

BANISH GUILT

When children come along, the work/life balance can sometimes get out of kilter. Life coach Kim Morgan offers her advice for anyone who's ever felt torn between being a perfect parent and pursuing their career goals.

Feeling guilty about something we think we should be doing differently is a pointless emotion. If we can't change things, then we have to change our feelings of guilt and accept the situation. Guilt can lead to stress and a feelings of powerlessness as we beat ourselves up and judge ourselves over something we feel we should do or shouldn't haven't done. Here's how to control your feelings of guilt:

- Forgive yourself for whatever you did or didn't do. If there is a pain-free way of changing the situation that is making you feel guilty, do it.
- Use a responsibility pie chart to change your perspective: draw a large circle on a piece of paper to represent something you think is your responsibility and that you feel guilty about. Try to think about the situation objectively. Divide the circle into sections, apportioning responsibility for the situation between you, other people and external factors. This powerful exercise will enable you to develop a more balanced perspective on situations in which you feel guilty, and will help you see that it's not all down to you.

THE ROLES, NEEDS, AND RIGHTS OF PARENTS

- First, make a list of all the roles you play as a parent. Then make a list of all your needs as an adult and list them under the following headings: physical, intellectual, social, spiritual, and emotional. What do you have to change so that your needs will be met?
- What will be the benefits to you, your partner, and your children if you all manage to have your needs met? Next, consider the following suggestions for the rights of parents:
- Parents have the same right as their children to be listened to and respected. Parents have a right to time for relaxation and self-development. They also have a right to time alone with a spouse or significant other. Parents have a right to postpone making a decision until they have had time to think. Parents have a right to say no and set reasonable limits for their children. Parents have a right to have their work at home valued by the significant people in their lives. Which of your rights would be hardest to claim? What can you do to change this? Who can support you?

GET WHAT YOU WANT—AT ANY AGE!

Yes, you can get what you want, even if you've tried and struggled to achieve your goals before. Put the past aside, learn from your mistakes and move on. Here's how to achieve your goals...

Getting what you want in life can be achieved at any age, provided you're willing to work hard to reach your goals. However, as we age there can be a tendency to become more cynical and less optimistic about life based on the fact that we've experienced some setbacks. But getting older shouldn't be a barrier to success. "Becoming older can be a challenging subject for many women," says life coach Anna Wilk (www. annawilk.com). "But there are examples of women who actually had their first successes later in life: Louise Hay, Grandma Moses, Susan Boyle or DJ Mamy Rock, to name a few. Older age can be our best friend, as we often have more experience, life wisdom and understanding. With age we become more confident."

Carol Boyce and Lucia Williams, weight-loss experts and co-founders of Vitality TV, agree that success can often come later on. "The first thing we tell our clients is that age is just a number, and it's never too late to write themselves a new story. English fashion designer Cath Kidston was a 37-year-old breast cancer survivor when she opened a shop selling her handmade tea towels. At 56, she'd become a world-renowned brand."

BE OPTIMISTIC

It's important to remain optimistic about your ability to achieve what you want and remember that setbacks are only temporary. If something hasn't worked for you in the past, it may be because your method wasn't right—it doesn't mean you couldn't achieve your goal. You can learn from that and change your tactics. Meanwhile, it's important to remain positive so that you have the motivation to keep going. If you feel like you're stuck in a rut, the best way to move forward is to start from the ground up. Carol Boyce says: "You need to make changes on the inside before you start trying to change things on the outside. Because if we don't change the inside we'll end up in another rut, no matter how many changes we've made on the outside. The healthier we are, inside and out, the more powerful we feel about being able to change our situation."

PRACTICAL TIPS

Life coach Anna Wilk says: "Start by answering this question: 'In what area do you feel stuck and how does it affect other parts of your life?' Once we map out the source of this stuck feeling and acknowledge it, we can decide what we can do with it. Once we make the smallest movement, the smallest possible action we can take to make a difference, we see the ripple effect. As the ripples spread, we might be encouraged to take bigger steps without feeling overwhelmed and out of our comfort zone.'" Anna suggests that you consider your personality type when making changes. "If

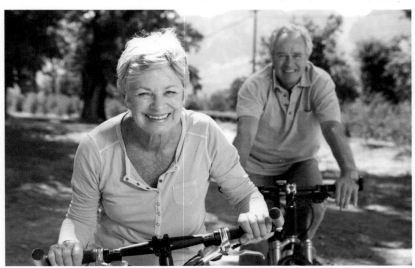

you think you have a more adventurous character, you may be happier making big changes," she says. "But, for many people, starting small helps them get unstuck at a comfortable pace, without jeopardizing their most important relationships and commitment." Figure out what makes you happy and how you can have more of that in your life, then make small manageable changes to your daily life.

KEEP ON LEARNING!
The famous quote from Henry Ford (founder of Ford Motor Company) sums it all up perfectly: "Whether you believe you can or believe you can't, you're probably right." Ford also believed that it's important to keep learning: "Anyone who stops learning is old, whether at 20 or 80. Anyone who keeps learning stays young."

Enlisting help and support from others can be useful, too. "No matter how much we believe we can do it all ourselves, how many talents we have and how capable we are, we need to work with others," says Anna. "You might try and do it all yourself, and that will work out, right up to the time when it stops working. Plus, it will be a very lonely journey. I've never met a person who achieved any kind of success without the help of others."

FIND A BALANCE

Remember, life is also about achieving a good balance between work, rest and play, so that you look after your health and have the energy to achieve goals. "Even if we love what we do, it's vital to create space where we are away from work, whatever 'work' might mean," says Anna. "Working long hours without breaks, holidays, or time off will create problems in other areas of life. We can easily lose ourselves and it will cause burnout and lack of motivation in the long run. Keep your work and life space separate, create boundaries with bosses and clients and schedule your work hours and stick to them. Find time for any form of exercise—and learn to say no to people."

KEEP A JOURNAL

It can also be useful to keep a journal of your progress to stay motivated. This means you'll be able to look back on what you've done and see how much you've achieved. Carol Boyce also recommends making a note of the good things in your life. "Start by making a list of everything you have to be grateful for," she says. "It's a powerful exercise because that list can include things like being grateful for having a safe, warm home to live in, or being grateful for your job—even if you don't enjoy it right now—because it allows you to pay your bills while you sort out what you want to be doing. When practicing gratitude, instead of focusing on the ways our life isn't working, we become much more creative about how we can make the changes we need to make."

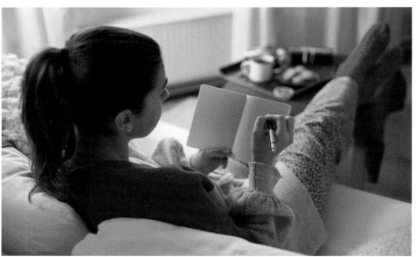

Left: Gratitude journaling involves keeping a diary of things you feel grateful for. You might write down something nice that happened that day, something you like about your home, or describe someone special in your life. You could devote a special notebook to the task, or you might also just type notes into your phone.

> **GRATITUDE MAKES YOU HAPPIER!**
> Gratitude can take many forms, from saying a prayer to writing notes in a journal, but whichever way you choose to give thanks for the good things in your life, it will improve your wellbeing, help you cope with adversity, and strengthen your relationships.

YOU CAN HAVE IT IF YOU
REALLY WANT IT!

Try life coach Jeff Archer's ideas for achieving goals:

• State your outcome as a positive goal—what are you aiming
to achieve?

• Establish precisely where you are now in relation to your chosen objective.
Be clear on how much work needs to be done to bridge the gap.

• Ask yourself, what will I see, hear, and feel when I achieve my outcome?
Establish how you will know when you have achieved your outcome—what evidence
will you experience?

• What will achieving this outcome do for you? What's the point of making the effort?

• Check that your chosen outcome is created by you and will benefit you.

• Establish what resources you will need to achieve your outcome—what's
missing in your current routine that will need to feature in the future?

• Be aware of any costs to you, or anyone else, of you achieving
your outcome.

• Make sure your chosen outcome is within your control
and that your success is not at the
mercy of others.

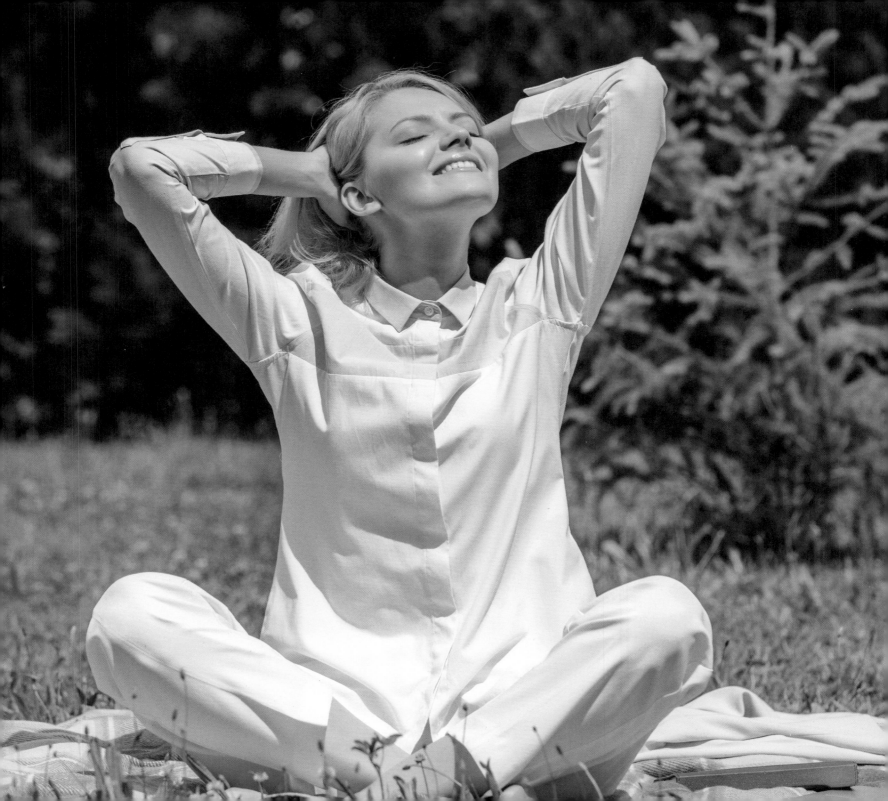

2
FREE YOUR MIND

Having good mental health means looking after your emotional, psychological, and social needs. This is every bit as important as taking care of your physical health, because the state of your mind affects how you think, feel, and act, and determines how well you are able to cope with stress, relate to others and make healthy life choices. This chapter is full of tips and techniques to banish stress and anxiety, and improve your happiness potential.

WHY WORRY?

What keeps you awake at night? Whether it's going over bank statements or paying a visit to Dr. Google under the covers, it's all too easy to get into a state of worry.

According to a study conducted by Rescue Remedy, 86 percent of adults consider themselves worriers and confess to spending almost two hours a day ruminating—that's around a month a year! And while many of us are comfortable sharing our concerns with other people, one in four keep their worries bottled up, leading to even more feelings of stress. "Most worry tends to have a particular focus – that could be worrying about specific people, situations or events," says Karol Ward, psychotherapist and author of *Worried Sick: Break Free from Chronic Worry to Achieve Mental & Physical Health*. "Worry is a very broad term, but it can be broken down into four categories: circumstantial (losing job, world events), chronic (always anticipating the worse-case scenario), catastrophizing (expanding one issue until we lose perspective), and anxiety (a constant low-level state of fear and nervousness)." Although a healthy amount of worry can be a natural coping mechanism, there's a fine line between a fleeting concern and chronic stress. "Long-term worry where people feel out of control and not able to do anything about the situation is harmful for the body and immune system," says Dr. Balu Pitchiah (emotionalwellnessclinic.co.uk).

"We often hear people say, 'I worry too much,'" says Professor Margareta James, a psychologist at the Harley Street Wellbeing Clinic. "Worrying affects not just our mental/emotional health but our physical health. It increases stress hormone levels, and it all kicks off from there." If it sticks around, something as small as a nagging concern in the back of your mind can affect your heart. It can make you more likely to have high blood pressure, a heart attack or a stroke."

> "Nothing is permanent in this wicked world—not even our troubles."
> Charlie Chaplin

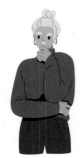 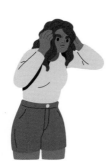 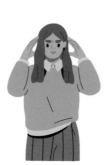 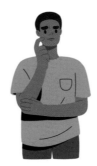 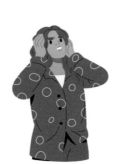 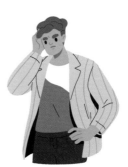 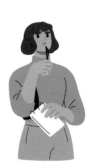

WORRYING IS NORMAL

Now before you begin to worry about how all your worrying is affecting your health, we're here to tell you it's completely normal to be concerned or anxious about things beyond your control. "Worry is rooted in our biology," says clinical psychologist Dr. Aria (dr-aria.com), who specializes in the relationship between mental and physical health. "The tendency for the human mind to worry about worst-case scenarios is actually an evolutionary hangover." So, if you've ever been referred to as a natural-born worrier, take heart in the fact that this is a perfectly normal attribute—especially among women. "Because women's stress response is all about the trend-and-befriend rather than the classic fight-or-flight, women will naturally worry about their loved ones," says Meg Arroll, a chartered psychologist. "Managing all these competing demands often results in high levels of stress, which exhibits itself in behaviors such as comfort eating, poor sleep, and anxiety."

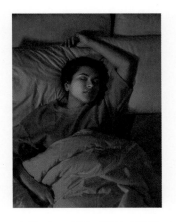

HELPING YOU SURVIVE

Historically, worry was a genuine survival method, designed to stop our ancestors in their tracks and force them to re-evaluate their movements. "If you were alive 200,000 years ago, worry could have saved your life if you were concerned a certain route across the desert was too dangerous," says physician, immunologist, and neuroscientist Dr. Alan Watkins (complete-coherence.com). These days, you could feel anxious walking a city street late at night. "This only becomes damaging if the worry persists longer than the perceived threat, and you start to generate higher levels of the stress hormone cortisol on a regular basis," he adds.

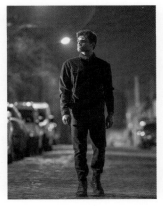

Although a surge of cortisol can be helpful if you find yourself in a life-or-death situation, long-term anxiety can suppress your immune system, leaving you vulnerable to more serious health issues. "When experiencing bouts of acute stress, cortisol is released and as a result the liver produces more glucose, which causes a spike in blood glucose levels," says Dr. Pitchiah. "In addition to this, your spleen discharges more red and white cells to send more oxygen around the body, which can lead to muscle tension, a dry throat and tightening of the throat muscles. Chronic stress has even been proven to result in heart problems, weaker respiratory functions, unhealthy sleep patterns, low energy levels, clouded thinking, weakened immune system, digestive troubles, gastric ulcers, changes in metabolism... the list goes on."

NOT ALWAYS A BAD THING

There are some people who believe that worrying can provide you with the right kind of motivation. "Worry does have a place in your life; if you didn't worry at all about things, you might let things that are important to you fall by the wayside," says Karol. "So, worry is not a bad thing per se, it only becomes detrimental when it keeps you in a chronic state of stress, inaction, and rumination."

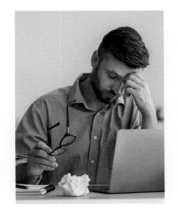

UNDERSTANDING ANXIETY

Anxiety has risen significantly since the COVID-19 pandemic, with many people drinking more than usual to combat stress.

In the UK, the Office for National Statistics says that the number of people reporting high levels of anxiety have sharply elevated during the pandemic. It's easy to see why. What we previously viewed as harmless activities, such as meeting friends, going on public transport, or simply leaving the house, now have a level of risk attached to them.

A recent nationwide survey showed that 70 percent of the UK population is anxious at the thought of being in busy places. Not surprisingly perhaps, 29 percent are having more unhealthy snacks and drinks than before the pandemic started. One in four admitted that they are drinking more alcohol. Couple that with concerns over finances, work, and family, and it's no wonder that more and more of us are experiencing moments or months of anxiousness.

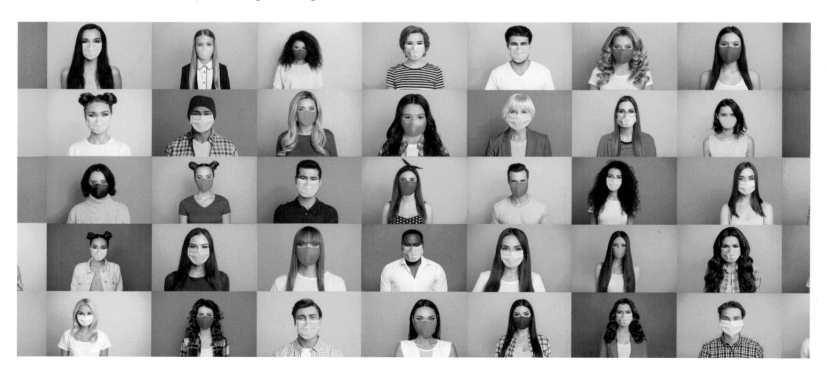

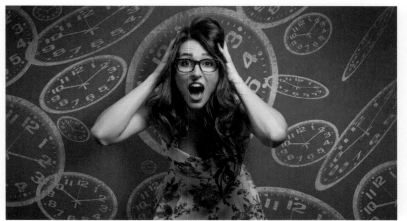

WHAT IS ANXIETY?

A racing heart, a stomach in knots and feeling on edge are all symptoms of anxiety. They're unpleasant sensations, but they were created to protect us. This "fight-or-flight" reaction is our body preparing to stay and face our enemy or to rapidly flee the scene. Whether it's fighting for survival, attending an interview, delivering a presentation, or lining up for a race, this hyper-alertness helps us to perform at our best. We all feel anxious from time to time. The problem comes when our body starts identifying normal things as a threat. When tasks of everyday life trigger these symptoms inappropriately or they continue once the threat has passed, this is known as anxiety.

HOW ANXIETY FEELS

Anxiety can be low and grumbling, creating a daily feeling of nervous unease and tension. It may also happen in sudden, intense episodes, often in response to a particular situation or thought. Anxiety sufferers may experience panic attacks, where a feeling of dread and fear results in hyperventilation, faintness, nausea, and heart palpitations.

THE EFFECTS OF ANXIETY

Anxiety affects both body and mind. Alongside the unpleasant symptoms of the anxiety come wider health consequences. In an effort to avoid anxiety triggers, the easiest solution is to avoid going out, however this can lead to loneliness, isolation, and depression. Self-esteem and confidence suffer, and life can become very limited. Longer-term anxiety is a form of chronic stress, which is linked to higher rates of many health conditions such as high blood pressure and heart disease. Alcohol excess, overeating, and inactivity—common with anxiety—negatively impact our health.

When your level of anxiety is interfering with your day-to-day functioning, concentration, and ability to sleep, then you need to take action. For some people, particularly those with pre-existing anxiety, this is an incredibly difficult time. Sharing how you feel and talking to someone you trust is a very important step. Alongside exercise and self-help treatments, opening up may be enough to help you move forwards. Help is available, too; counseling, talking therapies, and medications can all be accessed through your GP, so do make an appointment. Don't suffer alone.

TRACKS AND TRIGGERS

To understand what's causing your anxiety, keep a diary of your daily activities any how you are feeling. This will help you to identify what's triggering negative thoughts; once you know what these are, you might be able to eradicate some of them.

6 WAYS TO RELEASE WORRY

Take a look at our tips for dealing with worry and anxiety, and see what works for you.

1. Focus on what you can control

It is useful to identify any major worries and fears you may have, and then differentiate between ruminating and problem-solving—especially if you can't actually do anything about the situation. Determine what can be controlled and focus on things that can be influenced.

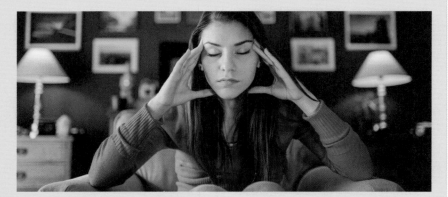

2. Practice gratitude

Write in a gratitude journal each evening—doing so helps you focus on the good in life, however small each thing may seem. It could be feeling grateful for a lovely, healthy breakfast, or showing appreciation for the friend you connected with today.

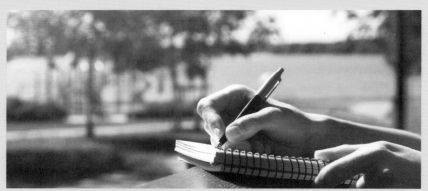

3. Live mindfully

Try to live more in the moment, which means being mindful of what is around you and your environment. Place sticky notes around your home reminding you to stop and breathe. If you take regular one-minute "time-outs" to pause and slow your breathing, it will become a healthy habit that keeps you more present and relaxed. Take action to deal with any problems you face, let go of things you can't control, and remember to stay rooted in the present as much as you can.

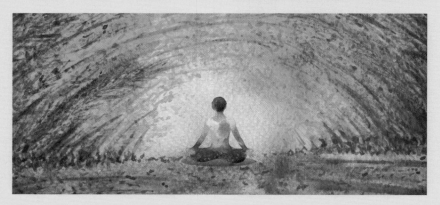

4. Do what makes you feel good

Focus on things that make you happy. Speak to loved ones (only if they won't add to your stress!), listen to good music, dance around, and watch comedies—laughing has a proven benefit on lowering stress levels. Or for a longer-term pleasure, do some gardening or plant some seeds in a container and enjoy watching them grow.

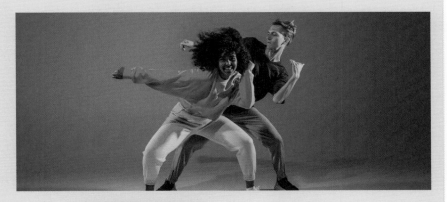

5. Limit worrying

Allocate yourself a set "worry time," perhaps late afternoon or early evening, after you have done your main tasks for the day. Set aside no more than 20 minutes to think over your issues and write something down about how they are affecting your stress levels. Write about how you feel in a journal, and then put it aside and get on with the rest of your evening. Getting your worries onto paper helps limit the amount of mental rumination that goes on, and is especially useful if worry stops you sleeping.

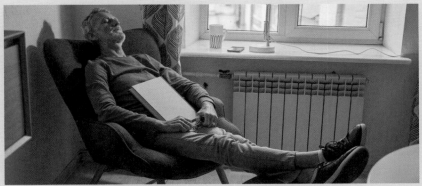

6. Try a supplement

There are herbal and other plant-based supplements that can ease anxiety and help you feel calmer. Cannabidiol (CBD) is proven to help lower anxiety and stress levels. The herb ashwagandha and the mineral magnesium also help your mind and body to relax and cope better with stress.

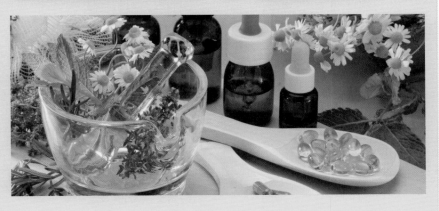

KEEPING WORRIES AT BAY

There are plenty of ways to get a handle on stress so that you spend less time feeling anxious and more time focusing on the fun things in life—starting with a little self-love!

In today's world, there's no shortage of things to worry about, from what's going on in world politics to worrying about COVID-19 or whether we'll keep our jobs and be able to pay our mortgages. Some people actually spend the equivalent of almost an entire month of each year worrying! In our books, that's one month too many, so here are some more tips on how to keep worries at bay. You'll find many of these ideas repeated throughout this book, so dip in any time and see what works best for you.

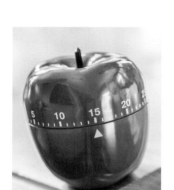

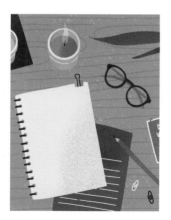

MANAGE YOUR WORRIES

Dr Meg Arroll provides the following suggestions for keeping your worries at bay:

- Create "good enough" reminders. You can use this phrase as a password (e.g. Iam@ goodenough), on a phone or tablet background, or a sticky note on your bathroom mirror or fridge. This will help you give yourself a break, increasing self-compassion and reducing damaging perfectionism.
- Fix your location device. When we worry, we tend to focus on events from the past or what might happen in the future. Yet we cannot change the past or control the future—we can only act in the present. To fix yourself in the here and now, "update" your internal location device by noting where your worries are situated—past, present, and future—then focus on what can be achieved in the present.
- Set yourself worry work. Plan some time for your worries. Set a timer for 15 minutes and during this time, worry your socks off! This will allow you to remove that background worry noise, so you can concentrate on daily tasks free from intrusive thoughts.
- Use tools to quieten a racing brain. A UK government-backed Good Thinking program (good-thinking.uk) offers a range of tools and resources to help you manage stress and worry. Or try the mindfulness toolkit from Think Well Live Well (thinkwell-livewell.com), which includes a 5-minute quick stress-buster.
- Write down your worries. Try to break them down into parts, ranking the worries in order of importance. Work out a solution for each task and when to complete it. Plan a reward for achieving each goal.

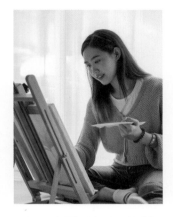

REPLACE YOUR WORRIES

Dr Aria suggests examining your worries and replacing them with more useful thoughts:

- Put yourself first. People often overlook their own needs, tending to put their children, partners, families, friends, and work commitments above themselves.
- Practice gratitude. We tend to dwell on absence—absence of a romantic relationship, of the body of our younger selves, or of the house, car, job, money, or health that seems to be just out of reach. Gratitude is the antidote to worry and dissatisfaction, as it makes you grateful for what is here and now.
- Guide your mind. Your mind can be your greatest help or hindrance. The secret to better emotional health is to realise that just because you have a thought, this doesn't mean it's true.
- Examine the worry. Is the thought necessarily true? Then, does the thought empower me to live a richer, happier, more meaningful life? If not, consider creating a more realistic, compassionate thought that leaves you feeling optimistic.
- Be gentle with yourself. When life is hectic, you can feel as though you're falling short in some way. Becoming less affected by worries involves giving yourself permission to prioritize your health and look after yourself, too.

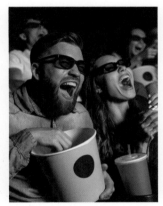

MORE TIPS TO TRY

Take up a hobby

Do something that brings you into the present moment through focusing on what you are doing. When you are painting, drawing, or creating, you bring yourself into the present moment and the worries about the future quieten down. Many people find gardening to be a similarly mindful activity.

Watch funny films with friends

Laughter releases endorphins—after a good laugh, your heart rate and blood pressure decrease, leading to a lovely, relaxed feeling.

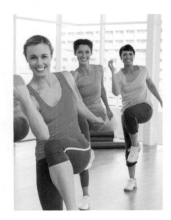

Exercise

Endorphins are released with exercise, and when eating certain foods such as chocolate and chillies. Doing a vigorous work-out gets your heart pumping, reduces worry and gets those feel-good endorphins flowing around your body. Studies also show that massage and meditation stimulate endorphin release.

CHANGING YOUR MINDSET

Here, Christina Neal, author of *How To Feel Less Anxious*, shares her top tips on how to combat negative thoughts.

It's natural for all of us to worry from time to time. Usually, our anxious thoughts will pass, or the everyday things that have caused concern will work themselves out in the end. However, constant worrying or feeling fearful for much of the time could be a sign of anxiety. As we've discussed, it's important to address anxiety and worry, because they can have a detrimental effect on our health in the long term. Before the COVID lockdown started, The World Health Organization (WHO) reported that one in 13 people globally suffers from anxiety. But even though it can seem frightening at the time, worry and anxiety can be controlled.

ACCEPT HOW YOU'RE FEELING

If you feel anxiety setting in, don't try to convince yourself it's not happening. Allow your feelings to wash over you. Repeat affirmations that may make you feel better or remind yourself of other occasions when you managed to get through this.

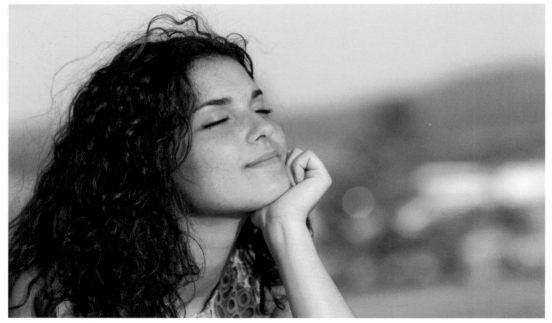

THOUGHTS ARE JUST THOUGHTS

Remember that negative thoughts are just that, and not necessarily facts or based on what might actually happen. Next time a negative thought creeps in, write it down, read it back and question whether or not it's really true.

Left: *If you find yourself thinking a negative thought, pause for a moment. Try to label your thought, using a sentence such as "I am having the thought that..." Create some distance between you and the thought. Then choose your intention. Think of a step—no matter how small—you could take to improve the situation.*

AVOID NEGATIVE PEOPLE

There is an expression, "You are the sum of the five people you spend the most time with." Notice how your thoughts start to change when you are around others with a negative attitude. Get them out of your life!

DON'T OVERTHINK IT

Try not to let your thoughts run away with you. Imagining the very worst possible scenario or outcome in a given situation is often referred to by psychologists as "catastrophizing". An example might be having a few harsh words with your partner and thinking you might break up. Letting your mind race ahead and wondering what life would be like if you split up will increase anxiety, when really your partner may just need time to calm down.

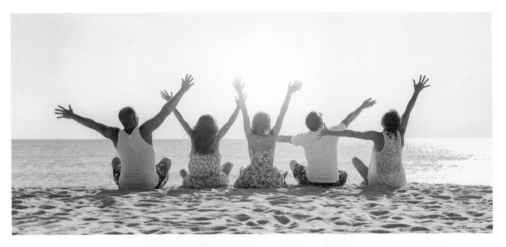

DON'T TRY TO MULTI-TASK

Multi-tasking will overwhelm a busy mind. Make a short list of tasks to complete and focus on one at a time. Close your email inbox while you finish a task, put your phone on silent and avoid digital distractions. Cross each task off the list as you complete it. This will give you a sense of control again.

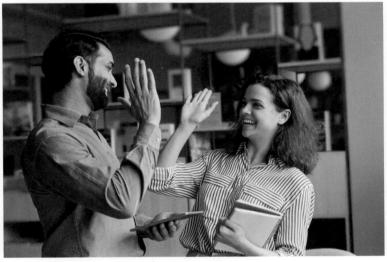

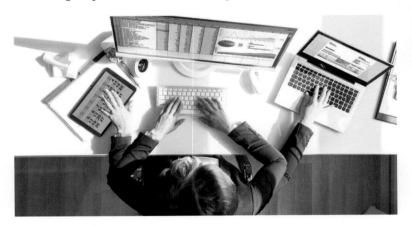

KNOW WHAT YOU STAND FOR

Look at your values and beliefs and see if they are being compromised. Your values are long-lasting beliefs about what is important to you. A belief is an idea that you hold as being true. You might be doing a job that goes against your principles, making you feel like you're putting on a mask and not being you. If so, you might want to consider changing your job.

TAKE BACK CONTROL

Regaining control of stressful situations, even if you can't get rid of them completely, will help you feel positive and more able to cope.

Physical symptoms of stress include headaches, muscle tension or pain, chest pain, fatigue, stomach upsets, and sleep problems. Your mood will also be affected. You may suffer from anxiety, feel restless, lack motivation, and be irritable and angry a lot of the time. Or you may feel sad and depressed. This can magnify itself in other ways—if you're trying to get in shape, you may be frustrated by the fact that you're tempted to overeat—or you may lose your appetite completely. You might drink too much or become more withdrawn socially. Stress is simply not good for mind or the body. But how do you deal with it?

Below: You can't control stress, but you can choose how you respond to it.

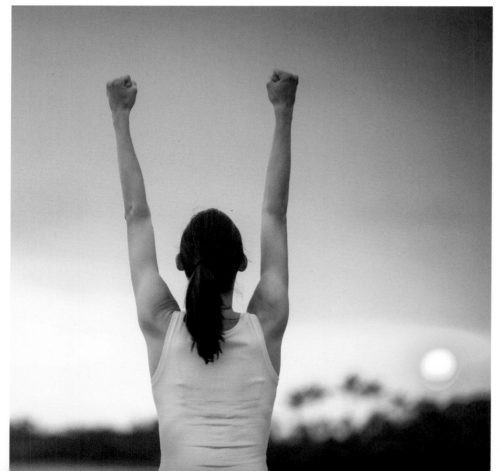

COMBAT STRESS

The solution depends partly on what is causing you to be stressed in the first place. Face up to the situation and have a careful think about what you can do, if anything, to combat your stress. If it's work-related, such as a heavy workload, you may be able to resolve the situation by talking to your boss. If you've already tried that and it didn't change anything, it could be time to change jobs. Or you could try to change your attitude. That may sound quite daunting, but do your best, as it can be quite a liberating method of coping. Of course, this may be easier for some people, while others may find it impossible to do. Another way to reduce stress is to try to take control. If you can't change jobs and your boss doesn't understand or appreciate your heavy workload, make sure you don't take on stress in other areas of your life. Don't let others burden you with their problems—have your own personal boundaries. Let people know you're dealing with a lot at work, and you need to relax during your

DON'T PUNISH YOURSELF

When you're stressed, anxious, or have a lot on your plate, it can be tempting to drink more alcohol or overeat. But Alison Cullen, nutritional therapist from A. Vogel, warns against punishing yourself further in this way—it won't get rid of stress and will only make you more depressed.

- Don't let the pressure tip you into self-destructive behavior that you mistakenly see as a coping mechanism, e.g., alcohol, smoking, or a caffeine-and-chocolate-based strategy. Set up some good habits, such as drinking a daily minimum amount of water, having a maximum amount of caffeine, and doing a weekly shop that provides plenty of nutritious nibbles and treats.
- Prioritize sleep. Sleep permits physical and psychological repair work that makes it possible to function well during the day, even under pressure. Gentle exercise will help burn off the extra cortisol, and structured breathing exercises can help calm you down.
- Know when to stop—most of us only discover our limits when we fall to our knees and can't get up. Being aware of how stress affects our bodies and taking preventative action can avert a huge amount of misery and pain, as well as save you the time, money, and angst involved in putting your nervous system back together again.
- Just say no! You may feel it shows what a tough cookie you are when you take on that extra work assignment or push yourself to do another gym session when your body is begging for sleep, but you won't feel so clever when your immune function hits the floor, or your memory refuses to bring up the simplest information such as your child's birthdate!

downtime. If stress is caused by something you can't change, such as caring for a sick partner or elderly relative, then take control of the situation as much as possible.

You can't control the stress, but you can choose how you respond to it—and how much you let it take over your life. You can also control your own health. By looking after yourself, by doing regular exercise (even if it's just for short periods of time) and eating healthily, as well as getting a good night's sleep, you will be better placed to cope with stress. It's also important to have some time for yourself. Many people use exercise as valuable "me time." Whether it's going out for a run, taking up yoga, or doing a class that you enjoy at the local gym, pursue an activity or hobby that's just for you and not about caring for anyone else. It will be a welcome distraction from the stressful situation you are facing.

FIND SUPPORT

Think about who can offer you support. Whether you're facing stress in your personal or professional life, have a think about who can support you. Who can you talk to? How can you let off steam without harming your health? Who will be a sounding board for you if you're thinking about changing your life to get rid of stress? Have a couple of friends on standby who you can trust and talk to when you really need to think things through.

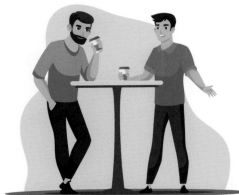

REDUCING STRESS USING THE "ABC" APPROACH

Focused breathing has been found to reduce negative emotional responses to adverse circumstances by around 20 percent. "A" stands for awareness, "B" is for breathing, and "C" is for compassion.

1. The first step is AWARENESS.
• Allow your worries to arise in your mind and allow them to pass.

2. Now BREATHE.
• Take slow, mindful breaths, lengthening your exhalation. Research shows that taking longer out-breaths stimulates the vagus nerve, which calms your body and reduces your heart rate.

• Also try bringing your awareness to the physical sensations of the air entering and leaving your body.

• When you notice your mind has wandered, gently redirect your attention back to the in-breath and out-breath.

3. Finally, choose a COMPASSIONATE action, such as running a bath or speaking to your best friend.

IS STRESS DEPLETING YOUR ENERGY?

Feeling sluggish? It's easy to blame exhaustion on poor sleep or a bad diet, but experts warn that chronic stress could be zapping your energy levels. Here's how to keep them elevated.

After the recent years we've had with the COVID-19 pandemic, feelings of fatigue have been unsurprisingly rampant—something experts chalk up to the body's stress response. "Feeling exhausted is one of the most common responses to chronic stress," explains Dr. Cortland Dahl, research scientist at the University of Wisconsin's Center for Healthy Minds. "When we face a challenging situation, the body's nervous system mobilizes to respond. The problem is that we can't maintain this for long, so if the stress in our lives never lets up, our nervous systems simply cannot handle it anymore. This is when we start seeing negative symptoms, like feelings of [being] overwhelm[ed], anxiety, or irritability."

MIND-BODY CONNECTION

If financial woes or health anxieties are raising your blood pressure, remember that stress is the body's normal response to a threatening situation. The body goes into "fight-or-flight" mode, releasing cortisol, adrenaline, and norepinephrine (a naturally occurring stress hormone) into the bloodstream, which provide a rush of energy that readies us for action. Indeed, this can have beneficial effects. "Mild stress can actually be helpful," explains Dr. Dahl. "We have an 'emotional immune' system that functions in a similar way to the physical immune system—both grow stronger when they are challenged." But when stress becomes too intense or persists for too long a period, it can overwhelm the body's ability to cope and start to deplete its resources. "When the stress response fires day after day, the hypothalamus does not go back to normal but keeps messaging the stress hormones," adds Dr. Tim Bond, natural health expert at dragonflyCBD.com. "It can take its toll on our energy levels, constantly preparing us for fight-or-flight mode." This is what experts refer to as chronic stress.

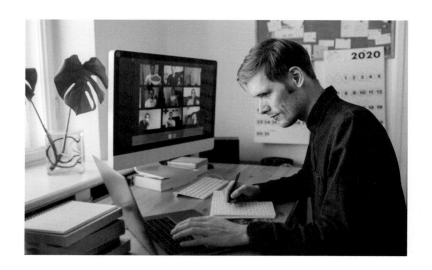
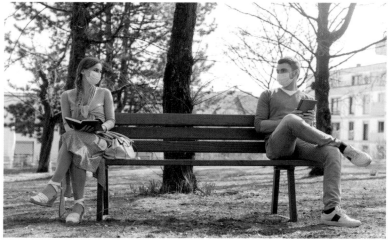

SPOT THE SIGNS

"Chronic stress can trigger tension headaches, worsen sleep, and it can lead to depression and anxiety. It can also weaken your immune system," says Dr. Bond. "The risk of high blood glucose, high blood pressure, low sex drive, and even fertility problems can all be caused by stress. "One of the biggest issues is that the symptoms of stress can create even more problems and weaken our ability to deal with stress even further," warns Dr. Dahl. "Chronic stress can disrupt our normal sleep habits, and this can make it even more difficult to deal with whatever challenges we are facing.

THE PANDEMIC EFFECT

While one in four reported feeling stressed daily prior to the pandemic, COVID seems to have elevated this to a whole new level. Nuffield Health data show that around 80 percent of British people feel the pandemic has had a negative impact on their mental health. The net result is that energy levels are at an all-time low. "The pandemic has created a perfect storm of factors that have led to overwhelming levels of chronic stress," explains Dr. Dahl. "Economic hardship, disruptions to our social relationships and work situations, and a tremendous degree of distress and uncertainty—there are few periods in modern history when we have faced so many challenges simultaneously. "And there's no sign of it letting up any time soon." Dr. Dahl says: "No one knows when or how this will end, and when the challenges we face continue over long periods, chronic stress can build and make it extremely difficult to cope." Luckily, we can strengthen our inner resources by finding ways to manage stress and keep energy levels high. A few simple lifestyle changes are all it takes, so try some of our energy-enhancing tips opposite and see if they work for you.

6 STEPS TO MORE ENERGY

1. Switch your sugar

A healthy diet can help to tame stress by boosting feel-good hormones. "White, refined carbohydrates won't do your energy levels any favours," adds Aliza Marogy, founder of supplement company Inessa (inessawellness.com). "Aim to eat medium- to low-glycaemic meals containing a variety of whole grains, vegetables, pulses, and lean protein. Eating this way dampens the insulin spikes, which can lead to energy troughs."

2. What supp?

Vitamin D deficiency is common during the winter months, and this can negatively affect energy levels. "A study from Newcastle University found that vitamin D is vital for making our muscles work efficiently," explains Dr. Bond. "It's thought the vitamin enhances the activity of mitochondria [the body's energy powerhouses], and what's interesting is that CBD oil can also help with periods of stress."

3. Stay connected

Try not to get overwhelmed by stress by staying connected with friends. "Making time for activities that we find meaningful will make a huge difference to helping us deal with the chronic stress created by the pandemic," says Dr. Dahl.

4. Drink up

"During the cool months, we often forget to drink enough water, which is important for keeping energy levels up," adds Amanda Callenberg, nutritionist at Bouzouki (yourzooki.com). Caffeine can elevate levels of the stress hormone cortisol, so it's best to skip coffee and opt for low-caffeine pick-me-ups, such as green tea. "Peppermint, chamomile, liquorice, or rooibos tea all count towards your daily water intake."

5. Hit the hay

Avoid the blue light that comes from computers, phones, and tablets at least an hour before slumber, and focus instead on relaxing activities such as reading. Stay away from alcohol and caffeine, and don't eat for several hours before bedtime. Keep the temperature of your bedroom cool, and close the curtains to make the room nice and dark.

6. Let the sunshine in

Natural light first thing in the morning helps to set the body's circadian rhythm by inhibiting melatonin production and stimulating cortisol. "Another good time to get outdoors is at midday when the sun is the strongest," adds Callenberg. "This can help your energy and mental function and lift your mood."

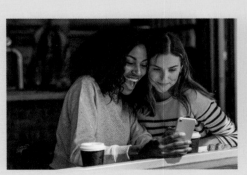
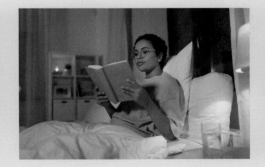
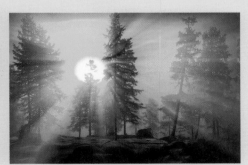

EXERCISE TO BEAT STRESS

If you want to get your stress levels down, then exercise is an obvious answer, but it's important to get the balance right and do enough to reap the benefits, without overdoing it.

The Mayo Clinic in the US lists physical activity as the top remedy for reducing stress. We know that regular exercise is a great way to calm our minds, but is there a particular frequency that is best for stress reduction? It is believed that those who see the most benefits from exercise in terms of anxiety reduction are those who exercise consistently. Try to exercise regularly at least three to four times a week. If you suffer from anxiety, it's worth noting that exercise can help to reduce your heart rate—and anxiety is often linked to an increased heart rate. Admittedly, during exercise your heart rate goes up, but as you get fitter your heart works more efficiently and your resting heart rate will be lower.

HOW MUCH EXERCISE REDUCES STRESS?

The answer is: not much! Your exercise routine doesn't have to be long in duration. Even just 10–15 minutes of exercise can improve your mood. A total of 30 minutes of moderate-intensity exercise daily is recommended, but this can be broken down into two or three blocks, depending on your schedule. "It is thought that exercise can cause chemical changes in the brain that improves your mood and helps build self-esteem," says Dr Roshane Mohidin, a practicing GP and behavior change specialist at Vitality (vitality.co.uk).

Exercise is also thought to help prevent anxiety disorders from starting. One study showed a 25 percent reduction in the risk of depression and anxiety disorders in participants over a five-year period. Chemicals released in the brain when we exercise can help us focus and deal with stressful situations more effectively.

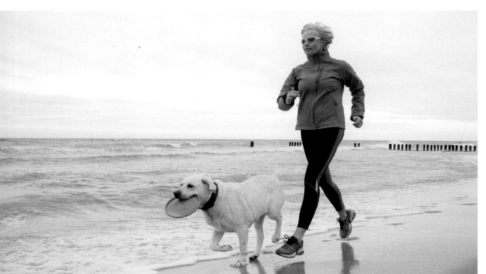

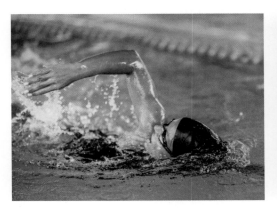 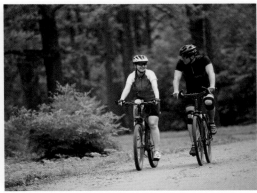 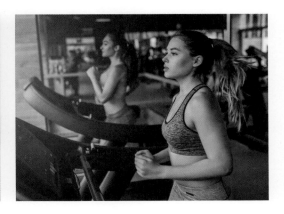

The best type of exercise to help combat stress are types that raise your heart rate. These include running, brisk walking, swimming, cycling, and using cardio machines in the gym, such as the rower. "While all types of exercise help with stress reduction, aerobic exercise is considered the most beneficial," says David Wiener, Training Specialist at AI-based fitness and lifestyle coaching app Freeletics (freeletics.com/en). "Doing exercise outside can also help relieve stress. Fresh air does wonders for the mind. It's way more enjoyable than exercising in a stuffy room." Strength training has numerous health benefits, but doesn't raise your heart rate as much, and therefore isn't thought to help with stress reduction. Yoga can help reduce anxiety, as it combines movement with meditation and deep breathing, which all help to keep your mind calm.

TAILOR YOUR EXERCISE CAPABILITIES

If you're not used to exercising regularly, it's best to build up your activity levels steadily and listen to your body. If you do exercise regularly, you can work out for longer periods of time, but this should never be to the detriment of your own health.

CAN EXERCISE CAUSE MORE STRESS?

It should be noted that too much exercise can become counterproductive. When we exercise, the body perceives it as a form of stress. This stimulates the production of cortisol, a stress hormone that is released when the body perceives us to be in dangerous or stressful situations—it's known as part of the "fight-or-flight" reflex designed to protect us when faced with danger. While cortisol is there to protect us from harm, too much of it for too long can reduce libido and fertility, and lead to storage of fat in the abdominal area. For this reason, a vigorous exercise session of over 60 minutes may be detrimental for some people. "The hormone cortisol, otherwise known as the stress hormone, has been shown to increase if you over-exercise," says David Wiener. "Performing high-intensity exercise for over 60 minutes a day can affect blood levels and neurotransmitters that can lead to feelings of stress, depression, and chronic fatigue. Stick to around between 30 and 60 minutes of exercise five times a week to get the benefits you need and also allow your body to recover."

STRETCH AWAY STRESS WITH YOGA

Whether you are anxious about a job interview, struggling to sleep or feeling burnt out from working too hard, discover how just ten minutes of yoga a day can help you feel better.

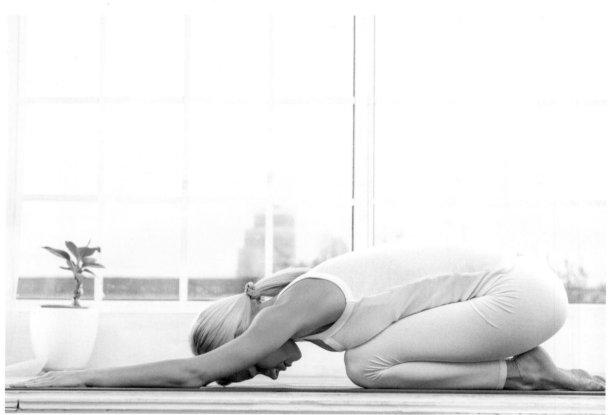

Many people start practicing yoga for the flexibility and body strength that it brings, but most will tell you that it's actually the benefits for their mind and wellbeing that keep them hooked. However tired, stressed, or anxious you are before you start a yoga session, you're guaranteed to emerge from it feeling renewed and soothed.

BALANCE YOUR BODY

Yoga has both short- and long-term benefits for your mental health. By relaxing your muscles and stretching key nerves that link your joints to your mind, yoga can have profoundly de-stressing benefits in just 10 minutes. Practice it more regularly and you'll lower your levels of the stress hormone cortisol, which is responsible for burnout and exhaustion. Yoga also primes your organs' repair systems, so your entire endocrine system is more balanced. One Swedish study reported that yoga was just as effective at reducing stresses as cognitive behavioral therapy.

THE STRESS RESPONSE

We're all familiar with the symptoms of stress—a racing heart, nagging anxiety, sleepless nights, feelings of exhaustion. Whatever the cause—a heavy workload, argument with a partner, money worries— if your mind interprets an event as a threat, this triggers a stress response in your body and activates the sympathetic nervous system (SNS), which is responsible for your "fight-or-flight" mechanism. Meanwhile, your parasympathetic nervous system (PNS), responsible for relaxation and calm, is suppressed by this response and your body is flooded with stress hormones, such as cortisol, which prime your senses and focus your mind, ready for attack. In the short term, this survival mechanism is just what you need to tackle a challenge but, on an ongoing basis, the fight-or flight stress cycle takes its toll on your body, leading to conditions such as insomnia, depression, aches and pains, and weight gain.

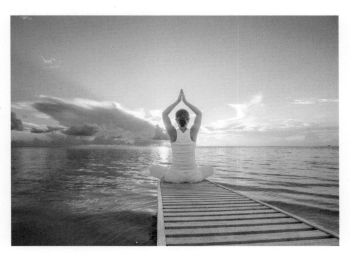

WHY RELAXATION IS KEY

Relaxation is a basic human need. Yet these days we often fail to give ourselves the essential downtime we need. But why is relaxation so essential? When you're working hard—physically or mentally—or you're going through a stressful period, your body releases stress hormones, such as adrenaline, to give you the energy to cope. However, if these hormones are constantly released into the body, they can damage your wellbeing by disrupting your sleep, playing havoc with your weight and skin, and eventually leading to burnout and accelerated ageing. One of the fastest ways to dissipate the body's stress hormones is to switch on your relaxation response.

HOW DOES YOGA REDUCE STRESS?

Yoga gives your body the tools it needs to respond and deal with stress in a healthier way, allowing your PNS to bring you back into a state of balance. One scientific study found that six weeks of hatha yoga increased activation of the PNS. Another study revealed that just one session of yoga can aid the nervous system. Many yoga poses such as Forward bend or Child's pose have a direct effect on your body's stress response, altering your heart rate, breath, and mental state. But in addition, learning to hold challenging yoga poses with a calm, focused mind and controlled breath helps teach you how to deal with external stress in a calm, controlled way. Gradually, your autonomic nervous system (ANS) imprints this response and allows you to harness it during everyday stressful times. Just as your body can learn a new physical skill such as mastering a tricky yoga pose, your brain and body can learn a new way to deal with stress. Practice yoga regularly and you'll soon feel ready to take on the world and deal with anything life throws at you.

LONELINESS AND DEPRESSION

One of the most noticeable fallouts of the COVID-19 pandemic has been the rise in loneliness and depression brought about by isolation.

Each of us has our own individual needs when it comes to social contact with other people. Some of us are perfectly content to live alone, while others prefer a more gregarious lifestyle. There's no "one-size-fits-all" when it comes to loneliness and depression; we all feel lonely or melancholic from time to time, even if we're part of a family.

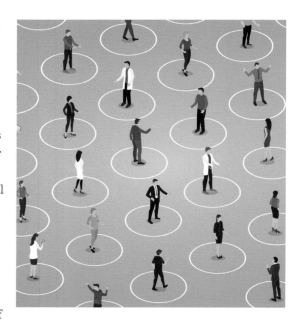

HOW TO BEAT LONELINESS

Here are a few strategies that can help with loneliness:

- Join a class or club with activities or interests that you like, such as books, cinema, art, exercise, or gardening.
- Volunteer for a cause you believe in.
- Strengthen your existing relationships by reaching out to friends, family, or work colleagues. Even connecting with just one person can make a difference.
- Adopt a pet. Animals give you unconditional love, which can really help with loneliness. A dog, in particular, gives you a reason to go out walking—and dog walkers love to chat!
- Talk to strangers you meet during your day, for example in a shop or post office.

WHAT MAKES US LONELY?

Loneliness has many possible causes, from big life events to changes in family circumstances or even times of the year. The UK mental health charity Mind lists the following reasons people may feel lonely or be vulnerable to feelings of loneliness:

- Going through a relationship break-up or divorce.
- Experiencing a loss, grief, or bereavement.
- Moving to a new area, starting at a new school, or changing jobs.
- Being separated from family and friends by distance or COVID restrictions.
- Working from home and feeling isolated from your colleagues.
- Special occasions such as Valentine's Day, anniversaries, or Christmas.
- Retiring and losing the social contact you had at work.
- Being unable to attend social activities due to mobility or financial problems.
- Belonging to a minority group and living in an area without other people from your own background.
- Having experienced discrimination because of a physical disability or mental health problem, or because of your gender, race, or sexual orientation.
- Having experienced physical or sexual or abuse.

DEPRESSION

Everyone has times when they feel sad or low. This is completely normal, and although it makes everything seem harder to do, the feelings usually pass on their own. But if the feelings last for a long time and begin interfering with your daily life, it could be a sign that you're experiencing depression. Sometimes it's not too difficult to spot the reasons for depression, for example in postpartum depression, where an enormous life-changing event has just occurred, but other times a downward spiral can happen for no obvious reason. Whatever the cause, depression must always be taken seriously; at its worst it can be life-threatening because it can cause thoughts of suicide.

Psychiatrist Dr. Diane McIntosh, author of *This is Depression*, advocates for more compassionate care for psychiatric patients and their families, especially given her powerful statement: "Every person, at some time in their life, will have a mental illness or love someone who has a mental illness." She adds, "labels like 'crazy,' 'nuts,' and 'psycho' have been used cruelly to describe someone struggling with a mental illness . . . The truth is, you can be 'crazy,' 'nuts,' even 'mentally ill,' and still be smart, funny, and articulate. When you're better, you'll still be a nut. You'll still be you, only well. By discussing depression thoughtfully, with compassion, scientific evidence, and, yes, a bit of humor, I hope to destigmatize mental illness, and embolden patients and their families and friends to stand up to ignorance."

WHAT'S WRONG?

"Depression is like a barometer: it tells us that something is wrong, but it doesn't tell us *what* is wrong... it is experienced differently by each person, so an individualized treatment plan is essential for recovery." Mary K. Tatum, mental health counselor

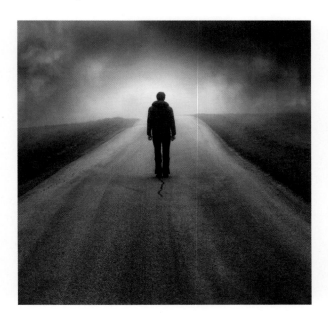

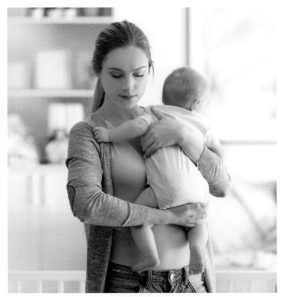

TYPES OF DEPRESSION

Here are the most common types of depression:
- Major depression.
- Bipolar disorder.
- Seasonal affective disorder (SAD).
- Psychotic depression.
- Postpartum depression.
- Premenstrual dysphoric disorder (PMDD).
- "Situational" depression.

12 WAYS TO HELP WITH DEPRESSION

Many of the ways we have already suggested to cope with anxiety are also useful for depression. Here are 12 methods that will naturally boost your levels of seratonin and dopamine, the brain's hormones devoted to happiness and reward respectively.

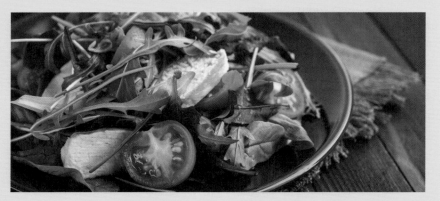

1. Eat a healthy diet

A balanced diet consisting of protein, dairy, leafy greens, and wholegrains is a good place to start. Or if you're vegetarian or vegan, you'll know that there are plenty of healthy alternatives to meat and dairy. Try to reduce your intake of high-fat, processed, and sugary foods, and be mindful of your alcohol consumption. It might seem tempting to open a bottle of wine when you're feeling depressed, but research shows that low feelings lift if you cut down on drinking.

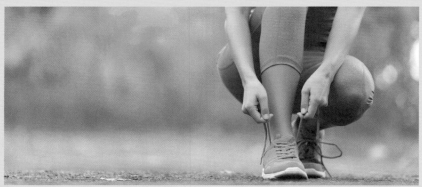

2. Keep moving

Exercise causes a cascade of health benefits, and we devote an entire chapter to it later in the book. Moving our bodies releases "feel-good" chemicals (endorphins), and these improve our brain function and can even work just as well as antidepressant drugs, according to Dr. Michael Craig Miller, assistant professor of psychiatry at Harvard Medical School.

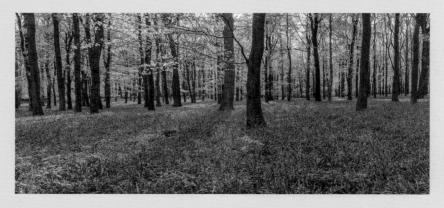

3. Spend time in nature

Being outside in a green space is a wonderful way to improve your mood, reduce stress, and lower your blood pressure. Breathing in the fresh air, feeling the wind on your face, and looking at the trees, flowers, birds, and insects helps you relax and get your mind back on track.

4. Stroke a pet

As anyone who comes home to the excited tail-wagging or purring of their pet knows, animals provide us with an immediate sense of wellbeing, joy, and connectedness. Stroking a dog or cat for 15 minutes is enough to prompt your brain to release more dopamine, according to research at the University of Missouri, Columbia, and interestingly, the dopamine effect is more marked when it's your own pet!

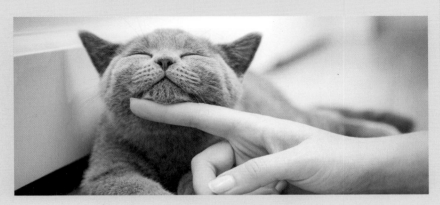

5. Swim in cold water

Weekly swimming in cold water can be an effective treatment for depression, according to studies reported in the *British Medical Journal*. The idea is that the coldness evokes a stress response, and your body then learns to deal with this stress. Swimmers typically report a quietening of their inner negative "chatter," followed by elation that can last for several days. If you don't have access to any outdoor water, a study in the *European Journal of Applied Physiology* showed that even showering for just 2–3 minutes in cold water can decrease the stress hormone cortisol by 34 percent and increase dopamine levels by 250 percent.

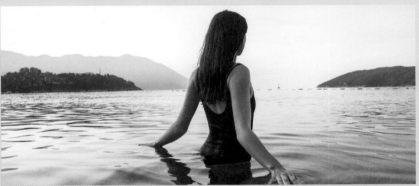

6. Talk to someone

Talking about how you're feeling is a really positive and powerful step in coping with depression. It doesn't matter who you choose—a friend, family member, your doctor, a teacher, spiritual advisor, therapist, or a charity worker on the end of a helpline—you just need to find someone who you trust, then begin a conversation. Being supported and listened to without judgement can be equally or more effective than any medicine.

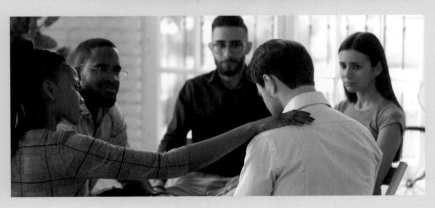

7. Go for a walk in the sunlight

Exposure to bright sunlight has been shown to increase the brain's release of both seratonin and dopamine, the hormones associated with pleasure and reward, and even spending just 30–60 minutes outdoors will do the trick. Soaking up the sun's rays helps with seasonal affective disorder (SAD) too, a form of depression associated with the changing of the seasons. And when you come indoors into a darker environment, your body produces melatonin which helps you sleep. Even in winter, going out for a walk is always a good thing, as you will benefit from exposure to vitamin D.

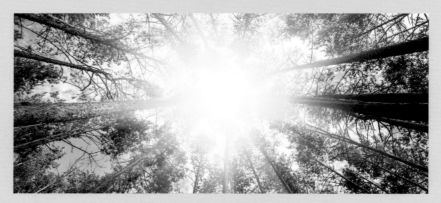

8. Listen to your favorite music

Isn't it uplifting when a song that you love comes on the radio? You instantly feel better. A study at McGill University, Canada, found that when people listened to their favorite pieces of music, scans showed their brains released more dopamine, and the chemical was also released even in *anticipation* of listening to pleasurable music. Further, attending a live concert has been shown to increase the production of oxytocin, a neurotransmitter that helps us bond with others.

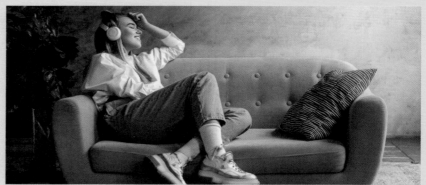

9. Make time to meditate

Numerous studies show that meditation has a positive impact on physical and mental health, reducing stress as well as lowering blood pressure and heart rate. Just one hour of meditation was found to increase dopamine production by as much as 65 percent in a study done by the University of California. Those who took part were experienced meditators, but the research suggests that even a short session can boost dopamine levels.

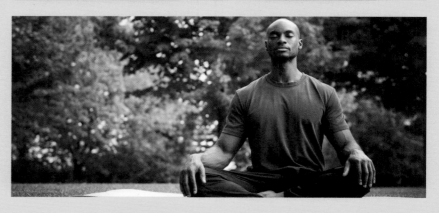

10. Book a massage

There's a long history of touch being good for us—Chinese practitioners, for example, have used massage therapy for more than 3,000 years. There are good scientific reasons why touch feels so good: clinical trials at the the National Center for Complementary and Integrative Health have shown that massage therapy helps relieve depression because touch releases hormones in our body that create a sense of emotional connection. So having a massage not only feels great, but it can increase your dopamine levels by 32 percent. This helps calm your mind and improve your mood, as well as easing physical aches and pains.

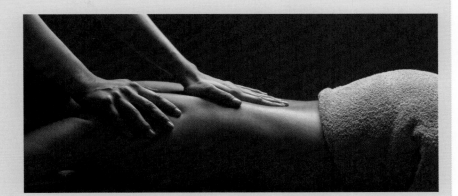

11. Do some deep breathing

The Center for Disease Control and Prevention recommends breathwork as an effective way to balance emotional and mental wellbeing. It reduces the body's stress hormones while oxygenating the blood and brain, and improving overall functions. Choose a special place to sit or lie down. Breathe in slowly through your nose, allowing your chest and lower belly to rise as you fill your lungs. Let your abdomen expand fully. Then breathe out slowly through your mouth (or your nose, if that feels more natural). Try to practice for 10–20 minutes each day.

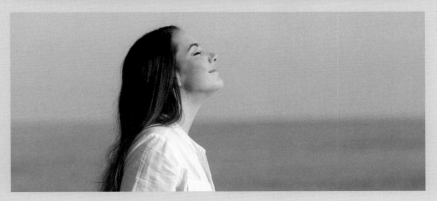

12. Stick to a routine

Depression can make everyday activities seem so much harder, but sticking to a daily routine can really help. In particular, it's important to get enough sleep. Go to bed at the same time every night, and switch off all electronic devices at least an hour before bedtime.

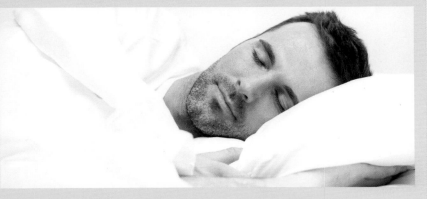

FOREST BATHING

For the ultimate mindful connection with nature, you might try forest bathing. The practice originated in Japan in the 1980s as a psychological exercise called *shinrin-yoku*, which means "forest bathing" or "taking in the forest atmosphere". The idea is to go into a wooded area and be calm and quiet among the trees while observing nature and breathing deeply. Forest bathing is a powerful form of "ecotherapy" that creates both physiological and psychological effects in our bodies. Here are some of them:

- Boosts health and wellbeing in a natural way.
- Heightens our senses and puts us into a state of mindfulness, in which we focus on the "now" instead of our "to-do" lists.
- Decreases feelings of anxiety and depression.
- Helps lower stress and reduce blood pressure.
- Provides an eco-antidote to our over-exposure to technology and city life.
- Helps people reconnect with their national parks and forests.

You don't have to travel to the wilderness to experience the benefits of forest bathing. If you go for a walk in any natural environment and consciously take in your surroundings, the effects will be similar. Be observant and look at the small details—the leaves, the branches, the ground, the sky, the wildlife. The colors of nature are soothing, especially greens and blues. Keep walking for a while, or sit quietly and take long, deep breaths. This will send a message to your body that it can relax.

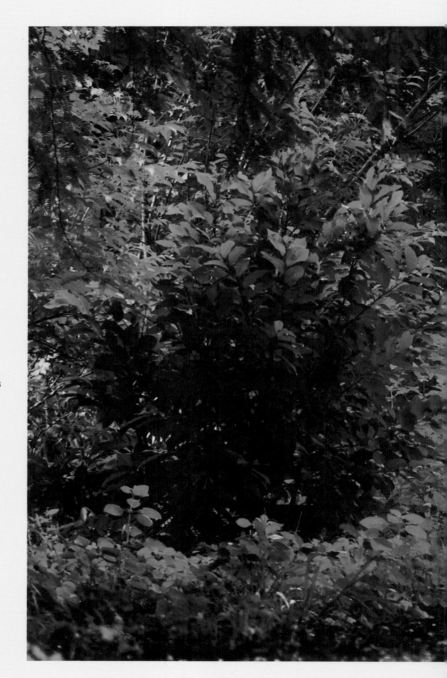

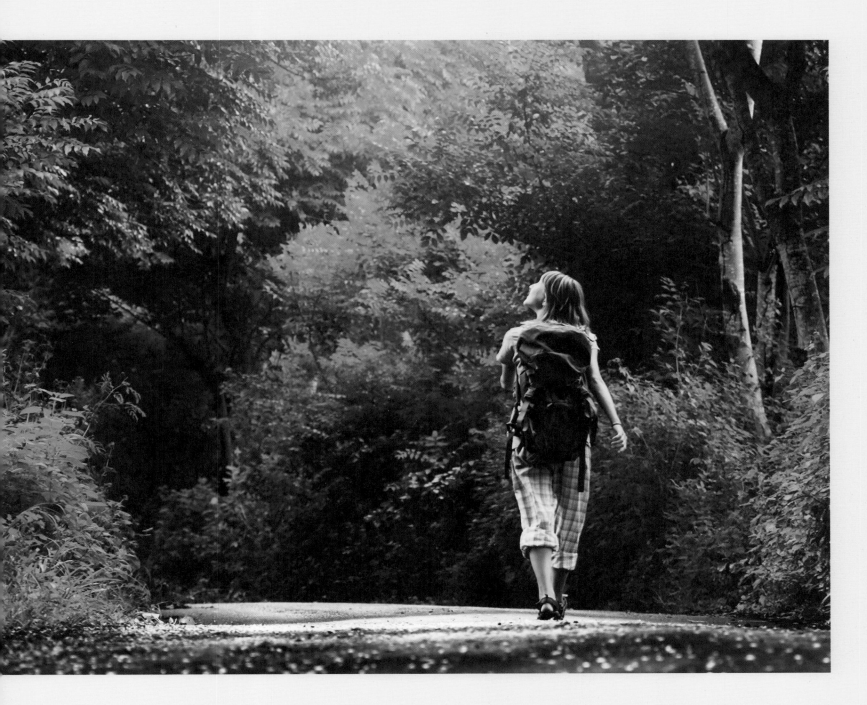

OTHER MENTAL HEALTH ISSUES

We've talked about anxiety and depression, but mention should also be made of the many other psychological issues and disorders that can occur. Treatments might include talking, cognitive behavioral therapy (CBT), or medication, in combination with the stress-reducing techniques provided in this chapter.
It can be useful to put mental health issues into categories:

• Anxiety disorders, including social anxiety, panic attacks, post-traumatic stress disorder (PTSD), and phobias.

• Mood disorders, including depression, bipolar disorder, and seasonal affective disorder (SAD).

• Developmental disorders, such as autism and attention deficit/hyperactivity disorder (ADHD).

• Obsessive-compulsive disorder (OCD).

• Eating disorders, such as anorexia, bulimia, and body dysmorphic disorder (BDD).

• Psychotic disorders, such as schizophrenia.

• Dementia, including Alzheimer's disease.

LET'S TALK

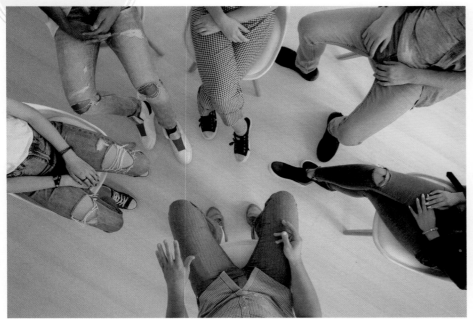

Many of us have regrets about things that have been left unsaid, and the past can weigh us down, but it's never too late to have that healing conversation.

Reenee Singh of the Association for Family Therapy and Systemic Practice (AFP) says it's common for people to want to talk about the past, but it can be more challenging for some families, in which case individual therapy may be preferable. Don't beat yourself up for leaving it until adulthood, adds Singh: "Silence can be protective and even help relationships sometimes. It might not have been the right time to talk when Abi was young, and it was possible for her and her father to talk later, when the issue had lost its emotional urgency. Some conversations need to take place in a reflective spirit."

INSIGHTS THAT FACILITATE HEALING COMMUNICATION

- Listening to others is as important as speaking. "When I work with families, it's useful to first set a few ground rules about how you're going to talk. This might include agreeing to take turns and not interrupt, react, or cut each other off," says Singh.
- Avoid the blame game. "During difficult discussions, it's easy to blame, but that can create conflict and hamper communication. I invite people to outline their experience and how they feel," says Singh. This also gives a sense of responsibility over our feelings, which can be empowering and help us move on.
- Being heard is powerful. Focus on the value of connecting, rather than outcomes beyond your control, such as hearing an apology. "A technique we use is 'active listening': People take turns to talk while others listen. Listeners then paraphrase what they've heard, which creates empathy. There's value in knowing you've been heard."
- For more information or to find a therapist, visit aft.org.uk.

WHY ARE YOU FEELING STUCK?

Your thoughts, feelings, and behavior may all be contributing to a negative outcome that prevents you from moving forward in your life. The good news is it's possible to change all of these, and you'll get a different result.

Identify what you want to move forward and write it down at the top of a page. Answering these questions will help:

- What do you hope to achieve? What long-term result will it yield and when would you like that to be?
- When you achieve your goal or resolve this issue, what benefits will it bring?
- What have you done about it before? Why has it not been achieved or resolved so far?
- What support and resources are you going to need and where could you find them?
- What would you tell someone else to do in this situation? List the actions you could take to resolve your predicament or achieve your aim—no holds barred. Which of those options are you going to take?
- What's the first step you can take and when will you take it?
- What could get in the way and how will you overcome it?
- What will happen if you achieve your desired outcome? What will happen if you don't?
- Now, on a scale of 1–10, how committed are you?

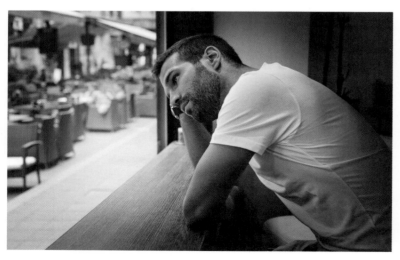
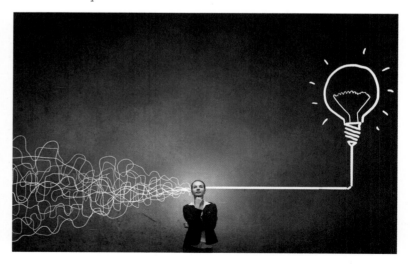

UNDERSTANDING
YOUR BEHAVIOR

Think of something you do well. It could be something you haven't acknowledged because it comes naturally to you: talking to people, selling, managing money, staying on top of your health and fitness, or being assertive. The thinking behind this exercise is that doing something well doesn't just "happen." There is often an internal program running in the background consisting of thoughts, feelings, and behavior that contribute to the outcome. Imagine if you had to explain how you do this to someone who didn't know how to do it. Answer the following questions:

• What goes through your mind before you do it?

• What do you say to yourself?

• What do you feel and where is that feeling?

• What thoughts do you have about the situation?

• Do you have any pictures or images in your mind?

• What keeps you motivated to do it?

• Why is it important to you?

• What happens in your body and your posture
when you do it?

DOPAMINE FASTING

Dopamine fasting emerged from Silicon Valley in the US. It's about temporarily avoiding addictive behaviors such as social media scrolling. Try the 7-day plan on the page opposite to beat hyper-stimulation and calm your busy brain.

Do you often find yourself mindlessly scrolling through your phone? If so, you're not alone. Data show that we feel anxious or stressed without our phones. There are other pleasures out there too: sugar, alcohol, shopping, TV. The world is full of stimulating activities that encourage the body to produce the feel-good chemical dopamine. But what if abstaining from these could help you find pleasure in simple things? Enter the dopamine fast...

BREAKING ADDICTIVE BEHAVIORS

Dopamine fasting was created by San Francisco psychologist Cameron Sepah, and is about temporarily stopping addictive behaviors and replacing them with seemingly mundane activities such as walking in the park. "The primary purpose is to spend less time engaging in behaviors that have become problematic," says Dr. Sepah. "The techniques are derived from Cognitive Behavioral Therapy (CBT), which is considered the gold standard treatment for impulse control disorders." Dr. Sepah adds that it's

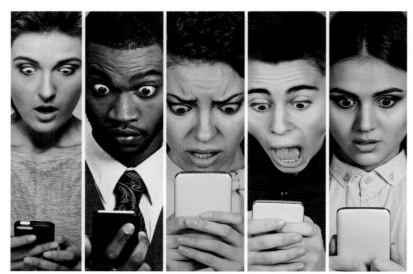

not about abstaining from enjoyment forever, but training yourself to regain control over impulsive actions. "You needn't 'do nothing' or meditate the whole time, unless you'd like to. Just engage in regular activities that reflect your values," he says.

"Dopamine activity spikes when a new reward arrives, such as food or drugs," says Dr. Ciara McCabe, associate professor of neuroscience at the University of Reading. "If you find certain behaviors, such as looking at social media, problematic, or end up watching endless TV, reducing your engagement with the cues could help you stop," she adds. "For example, you can turn off autoplay on Netflix, so you don't get cued into watching another episode." And many clinicians argue that the benefits go beyond dopamine changes. "It will also encourage quality interaction with people," says Natalia Ramsden, founder of brain optimization clinic SOFOS Associates (sofosassociates.com). "It will allow mental rest and, importantly, promote quality sleep."

YOUR 7-DAY DOPAMINE FASTING PLAN

Want to dip into the dopamine fasting trend? There are no hard rules. Dr. Sepah recommends avoiding all problematic activities—whether eating fast food, using the Internet or watching TV—for a block of time and increasing your "fasting" of these things over time, starting with 1–4 hours per day and building up to one weekend per year. Try out the plan below, but also feel free to include your own ideas, depending on your particular dopamine fixes.

DAY 1: Cut out coffee

Recreational drugs—including caffeine—are off the cards during a dopamine fast. Avoid them in the four hours leading up to bedtime to enjoy the added health benefit of better sleep.

DAY 2: Take a tech break

Give your brain a break from constantly scrolling through social media or binge-watching television by having a digital detox for the last four hours of the day. Read a book instead.

DAY 3: So long, sugar!

Dr. Sepah suggests either doing intermittent fasting or simply banishing unhealthy foods. Avoid highly processed products such as sugary or salty snacks for the whole day.

DAY 4: Start a shopping ban

Whether online or on the high street, give shopping the heave-ho for the rest of the week. Dr. Sepah likens shopping to gambling because it involves spending money to feel better.

DAY 5: Ditch Friday drinks

Just like caffeinated beverages, alcohol can be considered a recreational drug. Unwind from the working week with a non-alcoholic bevvy instead, of which there are plenty these days.

DAY 6: Be mindful of music

Some people on a dopamine fast choose not to listen to music because it can elicit arousing emotions. So, try spending your Saturday doing some quiet exercise, or do some creative writing or art.

DAY 7: Spend time alone

Natalia says many people fast from social activities, so spend time alone today. Try doing one of the health-giving activities Dr. Sepah recommends, such as reading, writing, cooking, or exercising.

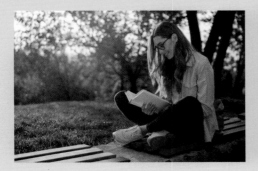
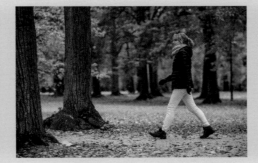
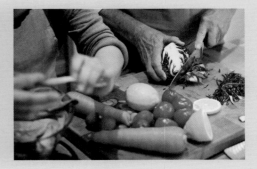

THE KINDNESS REVOLUTION

Embrace a new way of being loving by shifting your focus from mindfulness to "mindkindness," and feel the power of reaching out to those around you...

Around 2,500 years ago, the Greek storyteller, Aesop, said: "No act of kindness, no matter how small, is ever wasted". Centuries later, we are beginning to understand that never has a truer word been spoken, for the simple yet powerful act of being kind has far-reaching benefits. It has a profound effect on your physical and mental health—so much so, that kindness is set to usurp mindfulness as the route to wellbeing. When you are kind, your brain's pleasure and reward centers light up as if you were the recipient of the good deed, not the giver, according to research from Emory University. "This phenomenon is called the 'helper's high,'" explains Dr. Lorna Brocksopp, positive psychology and wellbeing consultant (joyfulsimplicity.co.uk). "Kindness has also been found to stimulate the production of serotonin, the feel-good chemical that promotes both physical and mental health—healing your wounds, calming you when you are stressed or anxious, and making you feel happy."

A study by the University of British Columbia asked highly anxious individuals to perform at least six acts of kindness a week. After one month, there was a significant increase in positive moods and relationship satisfaction, and a decrease in social avoidance. This is perhaps because helping others can leave you feeling stronger, more energetic, calmer, less depressed, and with an increased feeling of self-worth, according to a study from the Greater Good Science Center at the University of California.

Below: Giving and helping make us feel good. Studies show that generosity and kindness are good for us, lowering our stress levels and actually making us live longer. And when we feel good, we make the people around us feel good too.

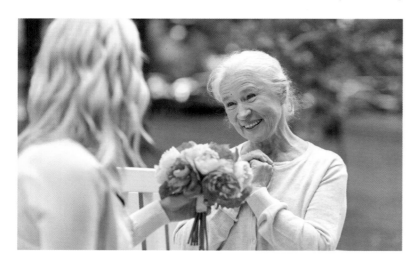

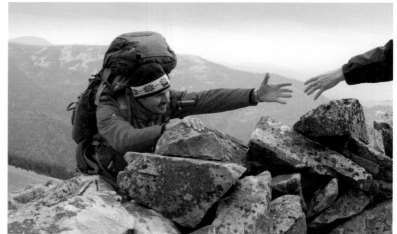

"Being kind and caring has also been found to provide a sense of empowerment and increased self-esteem, which is associated with emotional wellbeing," says Lorna. And helping those around you isn't just good for your emotional health, it's good for you physically too. "Research has shown that people who show kindness through volunteering tend to experience fewer aches and pains," Lorna says. "People aged 55 and older who volunteer for two or more organizations have a 44 per cent lower likelihood of dying early, and that's despite other contributing factors, including physical health, exercise, gender, marital status, and habits such as smoking. Helping others has a stronger effect than exercising four times a week!"

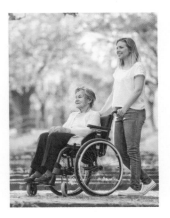

ONLINE ACTIONS

Today, some of the most visible acts of kindness are online. According to a survey conducted by the crowdfunding platform GoFundMe, the average Brit carries out 11.1 acts of kindness a month, including "liking" a social media post to make someone feel good, leaving positive reviews, sticking up for someone being trolled, and donating to charity. Indeed, our altruism has seen 50 million people donate more than £4 billion to campaigns on GoFundMe since it began in 2010. "What could be more loving than helping a friend, neighbor, family member, or even a stranger when they need it? At GoFundMe we see thousands of stories that restore your faith in humanity with their incredible expressions of kindness," says John Coventry, director at GoFundMe.

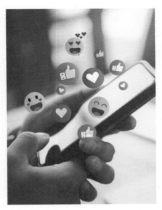

HELPING OUT

Kindness is also thriving offline. We still hold doors open for each other, take in parcels for our neighbors, and donate our clothes to charity, according to the survey. And 79 percent of women feel they are community-minded—with some going above and beyond. Kerry Lister-Pattinson, 33, wanted to help the homeless survive the colder months, so she set up Making Winter Warmer (facebook.com/makingwinterwarmer) with her friend Jo-Anne Burns, also 33, in their home city of Newcastle. "Winter is cold, dark, and long—and I have central heating and a roof over my head. For the homeless, it is brutal. That's why we set up our charity five years ago. We crowdsource everything from the 15,000 amazing members of our Facebook group. We collect warm clothes, toiletries, sleeping bags, toothpaste, and snacks, then distribute goodie bags across the North East. The people we help need a hug and a chat as much as they need a warm jumper, and we're happy to provide both. While there's a need, someone needs to help. We are both busy mums, but we will always make time for the homeless because every human deserves compassion."

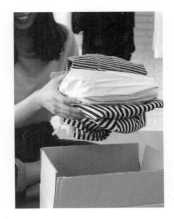

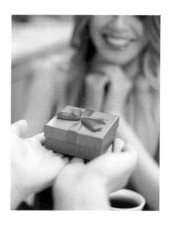

PAYING IT FORWARD

A global desire to spread kindness has given rise to wonderful projects, such as the Kindness Ninja Hut (kindnessninja.me). This annual, week-long challenge sees teams compete across the world to carry out tasks such as standing on the street with an uplifting sign, thanking someone who works for the emergency services, or giving a flower to a stranger. As the late Princess Diana once said: "Carry out a random act of kindness, with no expectation of reward, safe in the knowledge that one day someone might do the same for you." It's a powerful philosophy that still rings true. "Research has shown that the positive effects of kindness are experienced in the brains of everyone who witnesses the act, improving their mood and making them significantly more likely to 'pay it forward.' This means one good deed can create a domino effect and improve the day for dozens of people—kindness really is contagious," Lorna says.

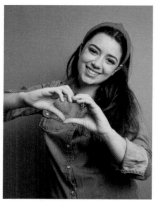

THOUGHTFUL IDEAS

Is there room for kindness in business? Charlie Williams, 45, and her business partner Lucie Carr, 39, believed there was when they set up their clothing, toys, and gifts store, The Kindness Co-op (thekindnessco-op.com). "When we sat down to discuss ideas, we agreed what was most important was kindness," says Charlie. "We promote kindness towards each other, ourselves, and the environment. Our clothes bear kind slogans because we want kids to feel good vibes. We work collaboratively with other small businesses and donate to the charity Young Minds with every purchase made. All the money in the world is meaningless if you don't pay it forward—that's what makes you feel good."

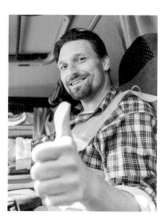

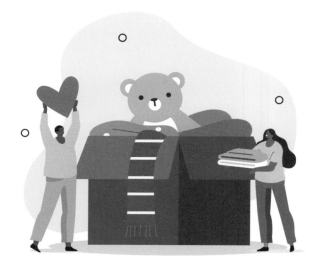

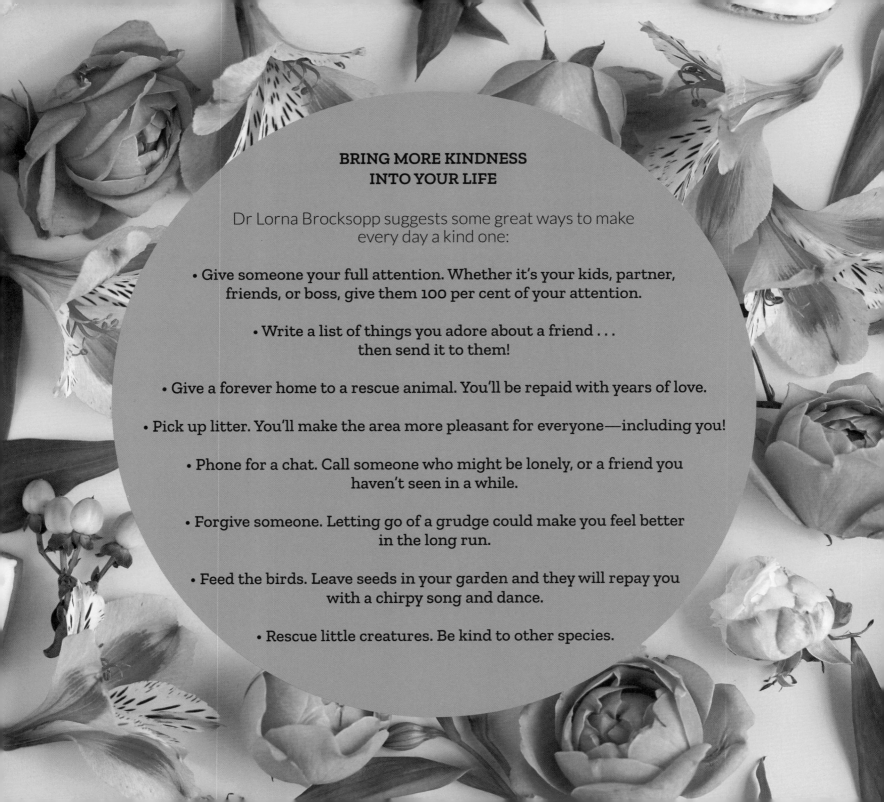

BRING MORE KINDNESS
INTO YOUR LIFE

Dr Lorna Brocksopp suggests some great ways to make
every day a kind one:

• Give someone your full attention. Whether it's your kids, partner,
friends, or boss, give them 100 per cent of your attention.

• Write a list of things you adore about a friend . . .
then send it to them!

• Give a forever home to a rescue animal. You'll be repaid with years of love.

• Pick up litter. You'll make the area more pleasant for everyone—including you!

• Phone for a chat. Call someone who might be lonely, or a friend you
haven't seen in a while.

• Forgive someone. Letting go of a grudge could make you feel better
in the long run.

• Feed the birds. Leave seeds in your garden and they will repay you
with a chirpy song and dance.

• Rescue little creatures. Be kind to other species.

HOW TO BE KIND TO YOURSELF

Self-compassion involves a range of components, such as self-awareness, mindfulness, and acceptance that we all struggle, and then taking positive steps to support ourselves in that shared struggle. Here are five ways to put self-compassion into action.

1. WHAT WOULD YOU SAY TO A FRIEND?

The first step is awareness. Think about what you would say to a friend who is struggling, perhaps due to a relationship problem or a difficult boss at work. You might give them a hug, tell them it's just a bad week, things will improve, and they are a great person. You may make them a cup of tea and listen to them… Now consider what you do for yourself when you are struggling. Chances are that you give yourself a hard time, expect yourself to get over your pain or disappointment quickly, and use self-critical language, such as "why do you always make a mess of things?" Do you see the difference? You wouldn't say those mean things to anyone else.

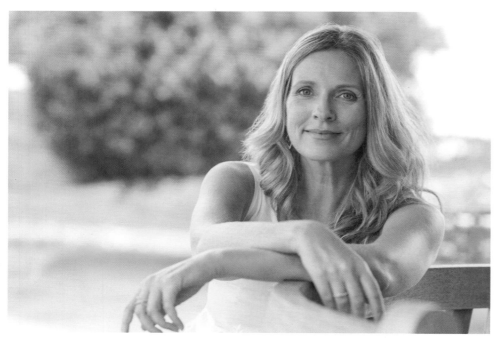

A useful tip when developing self-compassion in a difficult situation is to remember the prompt "what would I say to a friend?" then practice giving yourself support. This may feel alien at first, but start by making a list of the things you already know make you feel better—a warm bath, a cup of tea, a hot-water bottle, a walk in nature, a shower, a cuddle with your dog or someone you love… A common question that arises at this point is whether the list should include drinking a whole bottle of wine or eating an entire box of chocolates. These activities are about numbing painful feelings rather than soothing yourself. Try to stick to self-soothing methods that you won't regret later.

2. BE MINDFUL

The next step is to practice noticing your emotions and simply being with them. Much of our impatience to "get over things" is because we feel uncomfortable with our negative feelings, but if you can learn to notice your emotions and, instead of labeling them negatively, accept them and stay with them, you will move more speedily through the emotion. "What we resist, persists" is true when you begin to notice your emotional states. The next time you feel angry, try paying attention to what is happening and say, for example: "I'm angry!" and see what happens. The process of naming the emotion is calming and grounding.

A key component of self-compassion is mindfulness, which helps you stay aware, rather than being a passenger of your feelings and resorting to patterns of self-criticism. The self-compassion approach is down-to-earth: If you can manage a regular 10-minute mindfulness exercise, it's better than nothing.

MINDFULNESS EXERCISES

There are plenty of simple mindfulness exercises you can do throughout your day. Whatever activity you're doing, from brushing your teeth to washing the dishes, try slowing down and making yourself aware of your actions. Engage all your senses—sight, touch, taste, hearing, and smell—and notice the movements of your body. After some practice, you'll be able to apply your techniques to support yourself during challenging situations. Self-compassion involves building your own personal toolbox of these sorts of resources.

Make yourself a cuppa: Give your undivided attention to pouring yourself a comforting cup of your favorite warm drink.
Color in a picture or do some doodling: Just 5 minutes doing some drawing can result in a heightened sense of wellbeing.
Notice the everyday: Go for a walk and look closely at the trees, plants, flowers, birds, and insects around you. Breathe in the smells. Look up at the sky and notice the cloud shapes.
Do some deep breathing or meditation: Focus your attention on your breath as you inhale and exhale in a quiet space.

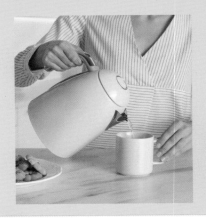 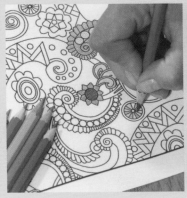 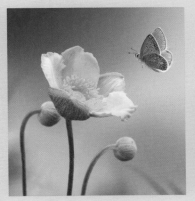 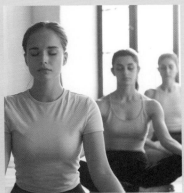

3. SPARK JOY

Another important ingredient of self-compassion is building our capacity for joy. You can savor positive experiences by finding joy in little things—a shower, a snowdrop, a hug. Practice gratitude every day in a journal and recognize that circumstances change all the time; everything is transient—good and bad—and even awful situations can offer self-development and opportunities. Research indicates that people who employ a simple gratitude practice report a better quality of life and are less likely to be depressed. Start a mission to grow your capacity for joy, one step at a time, by consciously noticing what you love in life.

WRITE A GRATITUDE JOURNAL

Brianna Steinhilber of everup.com has drafted a list of gratitude prompts that can get you writing about all the things you have to be grateful for. The following should be able to kickstart your gratitude creativity:

- List five small ways that you can share your gratitude today.
- Write about a person in your life that you're especially grateful for and why.
- What skills or abilities are you thankful to have?
- What is there about a challenge you're experiencing right now that you can be thankful for?
- How is where you are in life today different than a year ago, and what positive changes are you thankful for?
- What activities and hobbies would you miss if you were unable to do them?
- List five body parts that you're grateful for and why.
- What about the city you live in are you grateful for?
- What materialistic items are you most grateful for?
- Write about the music you're thankful to be able to listen to and why.
- What foods or meals are you most thankful for?
- What elements of nature are you grateful for and why?
- When was the last time you laughed uncontrollably—relive the memory.
- What aspects of your work environment are you thankful for?

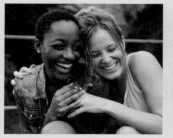
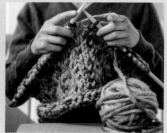
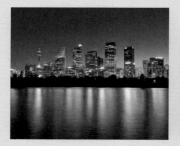
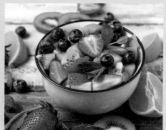
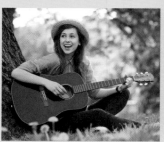
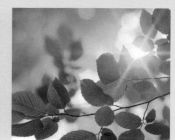

4. FIND YOUR INNER COACH

You might believe that your inner critic keeps you functioning at a high level, but Kristin Neff, associate professor at the University of Texas and pioneer in self-compassion, shows that our brain can't tell the difference between external and internal criticism. When you tell yourself "I'm an idiot," your brain experiences someone telling you "you're an idiot," which triggers a threat response. This obviously isn't a brilliant way to motivate yourself! It's more likely to result in procrastination, avoidance, blaming others, or feeling stressed and depressed. For example, how do you feel when you've scuppered your health goals by eating too much cake? You start criticizing yourself and, before you know it, you decide you may as well have more unhealthy food. Sound familiar? So how do you break the cycle?

The answer is self-compassion, which can help you change your inner dialog. For example, perhaps you want to eat healthily but slip up and berate yourself over it, which makes you feel bad about yourself. Using self-compassion, you might say to yourself: "I want you to change your eating habits because I care about you and I don't want you to harm your health. I know you want that too. What small steps can you take right now to get back on track?" Self-compassion isn't about letting yourself off the hook over something. It's about having an honest, supportive conversation with yourself—like being your own coach. It's motivating, not shaming, to be self-compassionate.

5. KNOW YOUR BOUNDARIES

Self-compassion is also about boundaries. Many of us say "yes" to things because we want to be helpful or a team player, even to the point of self-sacrifice. But this type of behavior can eventually lead to burnout, and it can be difficult to change it because you worry you'll be perceived as selfish. In reality, the outcome of having poor boundaries is that you can become overwhelmed, overloaded, and irritable, in which case people won't benefit from your self-sacrifice. Self-compassion is not selfish; it is actually a radical and courageous action. Learning to love yourself means you don't need to seek outside approval. You can be helpful without sacrificing your wellbeing. It's not all down to you.

Another concept to think about is equanimity: recognizing the interconnected nature of life and the limitations of our own influence. It's easy to assume responsibility for everyone and everything in life, and many people say "if you want it done properly, do it yourself," but the assumption that you are responsible for all outcomes and the purveyor of all the best ideas is a path to exhaustion. Self-compassion helps you to develop the wisdom to see that you can offer to listen and ask if someone wants help, but you don't have to assume responsibility, and many outcomes are beyond your control.

SOCIAL MEDIA BOUNDARIES
Setting boundaries is a good idea when it comes to social media. Limit the amount of time you spend online, try not to expose yourself to negative content, and always switch off at least an hour before bedtime.

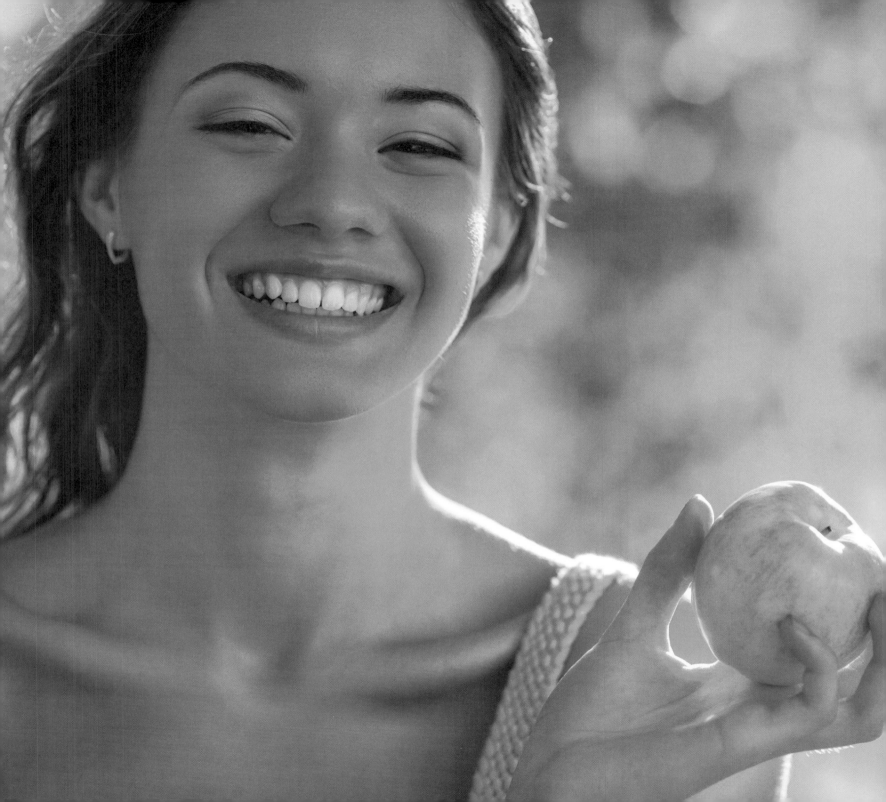

3
EAT WELL

A healthy diet is one of the fundamental building blocks of robust health. It's important to eat a wide range of foods to make sure you're receiving all the nutrients you need, and this chapter explores the main food groups and provides tips for revitalizing your body from the inside out—from boosting your immunity and beating stress to improving your gut health and keeping yourself at a healthy weight.

WHAT IS A HEALTHY DIET?

We all know the saying, "you are what you eat," and it naturally follows that if we want to function at our best, feel good, have plenty of energy, and live a long and healthy life, we need to think carefully about what we eat.

To function properly, our bodies need fuel from a wide variety of foods—and in the right proportions—so the key to a healthy diet is balance. The pie chart opposite shows the four main food groups in the ideal proportions that we need to stay healthy.

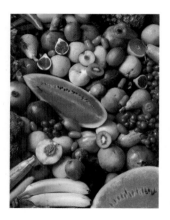

1. FRUIT AND VEGETABLES: These are a good source of vitamins, minerals, and fiber, and should add up to over a third of the food we eat every day. To do this, it's widely recommended that we eat at least five portions of fruit and vegetables per day. It's fine to choose from fresh, frozen, canned, dried, or juiced varieties, but limit your intake of fruit juices and smoothies to no more than a combined total of 150 ml (5 fl oz) per day, and choose those without added sugar.

2. STARCHY FOODS: Potatoes, bread, rice, pasta, breakfast cereals, porridge, yams, and plantains are good for energy and are the main source of nutrients in our diet, and should make up just over a third of the food we eat. It's best to choose higher-fiber wholegrain varieties, such as whole wheat pasta and brown rice, or when eating potatoes, leave the skins on.

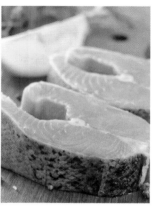

3. DAIRY: Milk, cheese, yogurt, fromage frais, and quark are good sources of protein and some vitamins, as well as being an important source of calcium, which helps keep our bones healthy. Low- or reduced-fat versions of dairy products are widely available, including cheese, so choose these wherever possible.

4. PROTEIN: We can get the protein we need from a wide range of sources and it's important to include foods from this group. If opting for meat, choose lean cuts and mince, but limit red meat and processed meats such as bacon, ham, and sausages. There are plenty of good alternatives to meat: beans, peas, and lentils, for example, are lower in fat and higher in fiber and protein. Oily fish such as salmon, mackerel, and sardines are good sources of omega-3 fatty acids, which help keep our hearts healthy, and it's recommended that we aim for at least two portions of fish every week. See overleaf for vegetarian and vegan options.

Note: Don't forget to drink plenty of water too! (See pages 98–99.)

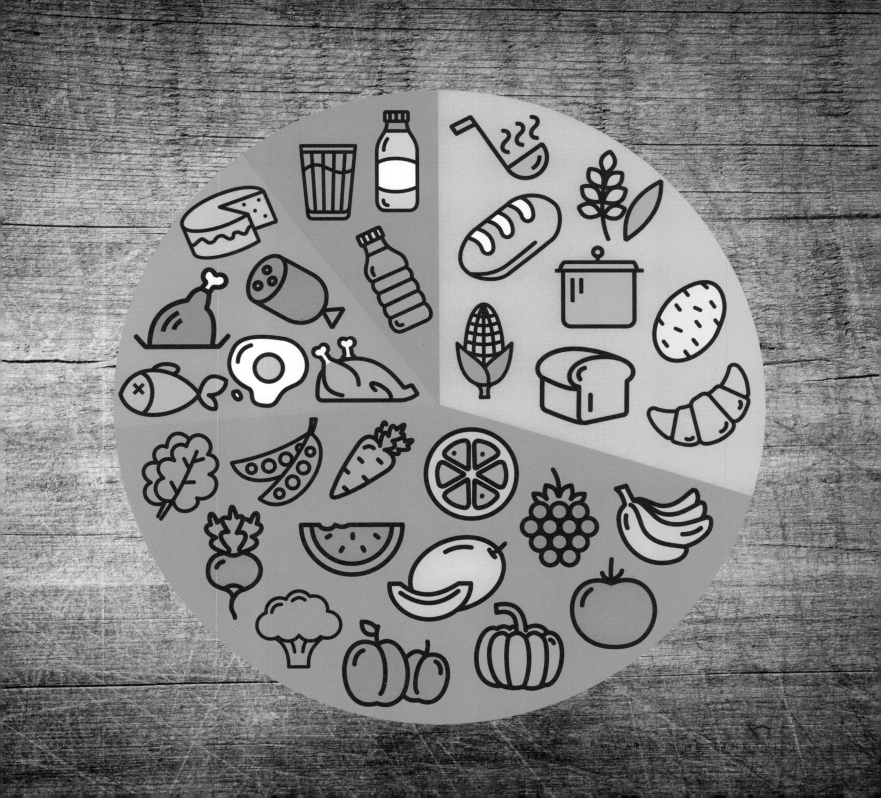

VEGETARIANISM AND VEGANISM

There are a variety of reasons why many people opt for a diet without meat. Some have concerns about animal rights and animal welfare, some have particular cultural or religious beliefs, and others try to eat in a way that lessens humanity's impact on the environment.

WHAT'S THE DIFFERENCE?

Vegetarianism has been around since ancient times. It was particularly popular in ancient India, where religious leaders and thinkers promoted the idea of non-violence toward animals. With varying degrees of popularity over the next few centuries, the practice eventually became widespread by the 19th and 20th centuries.

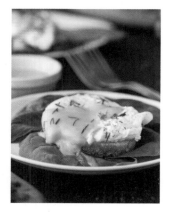

There are several subcategories of vegetarianism:

- Ovolactarians, who eat dairy products and eggs but abstain from meat, poultry, and fish.
- Lactarians, who eat dairy products but abstain from meat, poultry, fish, and eggs.
- Pescatarians, who consider themselves vegetarians but eat fish.
- Vegans, the strictest subcategory of the vegetarian movement, who abstain from all animal-based products, including dairy, eggs, and gelatin. Strict followers of veganism do not eat honey or wear products made from animals, such as leather or wool.

PLANT-BASED EATING IS GOOD FOR YOU!

There has been an increasing number of people choosing not to consume animal products based on their personal beliefs. But whatever prompts your decision to go vegetarian or vegan, there are actually sound scientific reasons why plant-based eating is nutritionally sufficient and even a way to reduce the risk of many chronic illnesses. According to the American Dietetic Association, "appropriately planned vegetarian diets, including total vegetarian or vegan diets, are healthful, nutritionally adequate, and may provide health benefits in the prevention and treatment of certain diseases." Here are a few key things to remember:

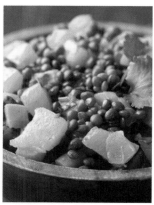

- Eat a wide variety of fruits, vegetables, and whole grains.
- Replace saturated fats and trans fats with good fats, such as those found in nuts, olive oil, and canola oil.
- Be mindful about nutrition and fat consumption, and plan your meals accordingly. A diet of soda, pizza, and confectionery is, after all, technically "vegetarian," but it is definitely not a healthy choice!

Have a look at the table opposite to make sure you're on the right track.

HEALTHY EATING FOR VEGETARIANS

For vegetarians who eat dairy products and eggs, a healthy diet is the same as for anyone else, but without meat, poultry, or fish:

- Fruit and vegetables should be the main part of a vegetarian diet, and you should aim to eat five portions per day. This includes fresh, frozen, canned, dried, or juiced varieties (preferably unsweetened).
- Starchy carbohydrates such as potatoes, bread, cereals, rice, and pasta should make up just over a third of the food you eat. Where possible, choose wholegrain varieties.
- Dairy or dairy alternatives provide essential calcium. This includes milk, cheese, yogurt, soya, rice, and oat drinks.To make healthier choices, go for lower-fat milk and dairy foods. Also choose lower-sugar options.
- Beans, pulses, eggs, nuts, and other sources of protein are particularly important for people who don't get protein by eating meat, fish, or dairy products. Meat alternatives include tofu, mycoprotein (such as Quorn), textured vegetable protein, and tempeh. You need to eat a variety of different sources of protein to get the right mixture of amino acids, which are used to build and repair the body's cells.
- Unsaturated oils and spreads include vegetable, rapeseed, olive, and sunflower oils, which are healthier than saturated fats (such as butter, lard, and ghee). However, all types of fat should be eaten sparingly.
- **Limit foods high in fat, salt, and sugar** such as cream, chocolate, crisps, cookies, pastries, ice-cream, cakes, and puddings. Foods in this group provide energy in the form of fats and sugars, but only contain a very small amount of other nutrients.

DAIRY ALTERNATIVES FOR VEGANS

The vegan diet is similar to vegetarian, but calcium—which is crucial for good bone health—needs to be obtained from foods other than dairy products. Here are some good sources of calcium for vegans:

- **Green, leafy vegetables** such as broccoli, cabbage, okra, spring greens, and kale are full of calcium, but not spinach (spinach does contain high levels of calcium, but the body cannot digest it all.)
- **Plant milks** such as fortified unsweetened soya, rice, and oat drinks contain calcium, protein, carbohydrates, and fiber. They each have different textures, tastes, and consistencies, so test them out to find which you like best.
- **Calcium-set tofu** is tofu made from soya beans and water, with calcium sulphate as its coagulant (curdling agent).
- **Sesame seeds and tahini** are actually much higher in calcium than milk! They are very versatile, too—sesame seeds can be sprinkled over a salad or added to a soup or stew, and tahini can be spread onto a piece of toast, used as a nutty dip for vegetables, or to make hummus.
- **Pulses** such as lentils, chickpeas, split peas, and kidney beans are nutritional powerhouses full of calcium, protein, fiber, potassium, and iron.
- **Brown and white bread** which contain added calcium.
- **Dried fruit** such as raisins, prunes, figs, and dried apricots provide natural sources of calcium.

Note: To help your body absorb calcium, you need vitamin D. Good sources of vitamin D for vegans include exposure to sunlight, fortified fat spreads, breakfast cereals, unsweetened soya drinks (with vitamin D added), and vitamin D supplements.

DON'T FORGET WATER!

Drinking water is often overlooked when thinking about wellbeing, but in order to function properly the human body needs about six to eight glasses (2 liters/4 pints) of fluids per day.

If your energy levels are low and are you finding that you're struggling to concentrate on key tasks, you may not be drinking enough water. In the UK, for example, nine out of ten people are not drinking the recommended six to eight glasses of fluids per day, and 20 percent admit they forget to drink water altogether! With our bodies consisting of around 70 percent water, ensuring we are sufficiently hydrated throughout the day with good-quality H_2O is essential for our good health. Dr. Naomi Newman-Beinart reveals some possible signs of dehydration:

- **Headaches:** Drinking enough water has been shown to help alleviate mild headaches.
- **Difficulty concentrating:** Being dehydrated can make it hard to focus, making your working and home life much harder work than they need to be. Reaching for a bottle of water is an easy fix.

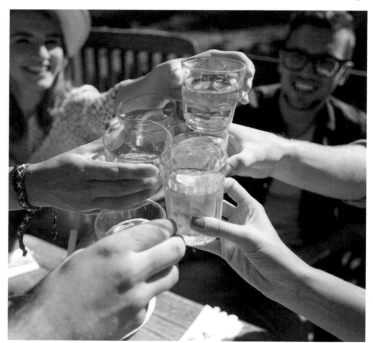

- **Low energy and low mood:** Even mild dehydration can make you feel low. Keep a bottle of water next to you as a reminder to take a sip every now and again.
- **Constipation:** Drinking water is an easy remedy for constipation. You may need more fiber and exercise, but always start with the simplest solution.

Hydration is needed for everything in our body to work well, from digestion and heart function to temperature control and for our brain to work properly. It is, without question, the single most essential component of the human body.

OTHER DRINKS

As well as water, you can also increase your fluid intake with milk, sugar-free drinks, soup, tea, and coffee, but note that caffeinated drinks can make the body produce urine more quickly, which has a dehydrating effect. Some fruit and veg can also contribute to our fluid intake, such as melon, courgette (zucchini), or cucumber.

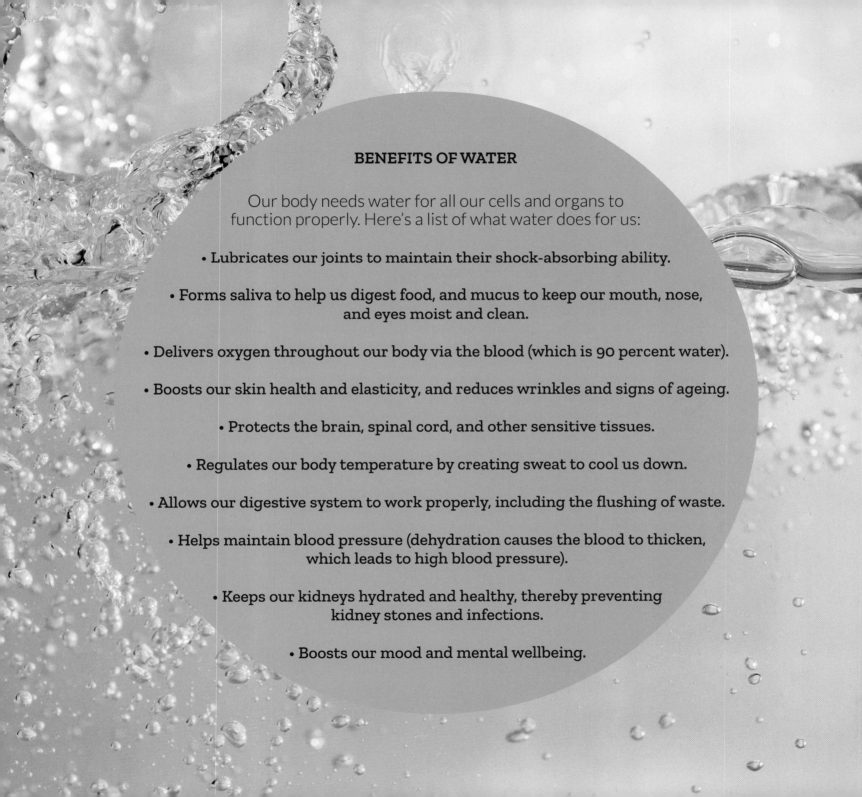

BENEFITS OF WATER

Our body needs water for all our cells and organs to function properly. Here's a list of what water does for us:

- Lubricates our joints to maintain their shock-absorbing ability.

- Forms saliva to help us digest food, and mucus to keep our mouth, nose, and eyes moist and clean.

- Delivers oxygen throughout our body via the blood (which is 90 percent water).

- Boosts our skin health and elasticity, and reduces wrinkles and signs of ageing.

- Protects the brain, spinal cord, and other sensitive tissues.

- Regulates our body temperature by creating sweat to cool us down.

- Allows our digestive system to work properly, including the flushing of waste.

- Helps maintain blood pressure (dehydration causes the blood to thicken, which leads to high blood pressure).

- Keeps our kidneys hydrated and healthy, thereby preventing kidney stones and infections.

- Boosts our mood and mental wellbeing.

10 WAYS TO BOOST YOUR IMMUNITY

A strong immune system can ensure your body naturally fights off any viruses and other pathogens that come its way. These nutrition ideas will help you stay right as rain.

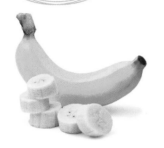

1. REPLENISH YOUR ELECTROLYTES

Electrolytes are tiny charged mineral particles that dissolve in your body's fluids and help conduct electricity. They are responsible for many processes, one of which is maintaining normal immune function. Some of the better-known electrolytes include calcium, sodium, magnesium, and potassium. For an immediate boost as well as long-term immunity, consume plenty of electrolyte-rich foods such as bananas, pickles, and coconut water, or a restorative salts solution, especially if you have recently been ill or you have undertaken extreme exercise. Calcium- and magnesium-rich foods include dairy, green leafy vegetables, and nuts. Potassium is found in sweet potatoes and avocados, and a simple banana is an electrolyte powerhouse packed with potassium, magnesium, sodium, and chloride.

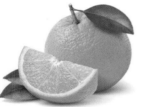

2. TAKE VITAMIN C

When you are deficient in vitamin C, your immune system doesn't respond quickly to invading pathogens. Vitamin and orthomolecular expert Andrew Saul (doctoryourself.com) recommends taking 5–6,000 mg a day of vitamin C, and up to 18,000 mg a day if you get a virus.

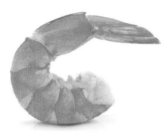

3. AND ZINC TOO

Zinc is super-important for your immune system—just as much as vitamin C. A deficiency leads to dysfunction with your immune system as it helps reduce inflammation. It is also a major factor in enzyme function, protein synthesis, and wound healing. The mineral helps to protect against viral infections such as the common cold. Zinc has also been shown to have antibacterial effects in the body. Food sources of zinc include shellfish, lean red meat, turkey, quinoa, nuts, seeds, brown rice, tahini, oats, and eggs.

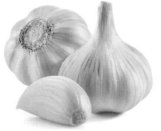

4. GO GAGA FOR GARLIC

Garlic has been used for centuries as a natural antimicrobial to fight infections. "Cook lightly to retain the active ingredient allicin or add towards the end of cooking," says Hannah Braye, nutritional therapist at Bio-Kult.

5. STOCK UP ON SELENIUM

The mineral selenium contributes to the functioning of your immune system. A lack of selenium reduces antibody production, making it more likely that a viral infection will survive in the body long enough to mutate to a more virulent version. Food sources include Brazil nuts, oily fish, shellfish, tofu, whole grains, tomatoes, and broccoli.

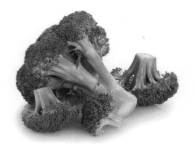

6. CHOOSE FERMENTED FOODS AND DRINKS

Foods including miso paste, sauerkraut, and kimchi, and the drinks kefir, kombucha, and amazake, have all been through a process of fermentation, so they contain bacteria that support your gut's microbiome. **Note:** Unpasteurized foods and drinks should be avoided during pregnancy.

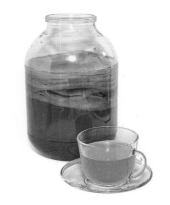

7. TRY TURMERIC

This wonder spice contains a powerful compound called curcumin, which is a natural anti-inflammatory that also helps fight infection and boosts your immune system.

8. MAKE A SOOTHING MUSHROOM BROTH

Mushrooms, especially the shiitake variety, have been used for centuries in Asian countries for their health benefits. Research has shown that this is down to compounds called beta-glucan polysaccharides, which may support the immune system.

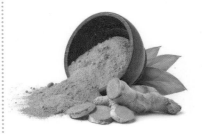

9. QUIT SUGAR

"Consuming high levels of refined sugar may compete with the absorption of vitamin C, which is very important for the health of respiratory tract mucous membranes and for maintaining the normal functions of your immune cells," says Alison Cullen, nutrition therapist and education manager at A. Vogel.

10. CUT DOWN ON ALCOHOL

"Alcohol can blunt your immune cell function by affecting the structure and integrity of your gut, where the majority of your immune cells live," says Alison. This has a knock-on effect to your liver, making it less able to fight off viruses. "Go for homemade delights such as pure fruit juice diluted with sparkling water, or hot elderberry juice," she advises.

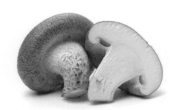

PACK A PROTEIN PUNCH

Proten is a key factor in keeping healthy—it is needed for the growth and repair of muscles. So whether you're a meat-eater, vegetarian, or vegan, it's important to get enough protein in your diet.

A healthy diet is made up of a good balance of fats, carbohydrates, and protein. Fat and carbs have hogged the spotlight in recent times, but protein is finally having its moment in the sun as we realize the crucial role it plays in maintaining not only healthy bones and organs, but in enzyme production and in keeping our immune systems functioning optimally. Protein is also a key factor in weight management, a topic in the headlines recently with obesity thought to be a major contributor to COVID-19 complications, particularly in the older population. Protein is filling so we consume less overall, making it easier to keep our weight under control. Another important function of protein is in building and retaining lean muscle. Muscle mass diminishes as we age—a condition known as sarcopenia—which can eventually lead to physical deterioration and reduced mobility. To continue living a full and active life, it's paramount to maintain muscle mass by eating plenty of protein.

YOUR PROTEIN-BASED DIET

And now the science bit! Proteins are made up of amino acids. Complete proteins contain all the amino acids our bodies need and can be found in animal-based sources such as:

- Fish and seafood (salmon, tuna, white fish, prawns/shrimp, and crab).
- Poultry (chicken and turkey).
- Lean meat (pork, beef, and lamb).
- Eggs.
- Dairy (cheese and yogurt).

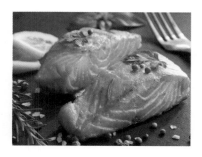
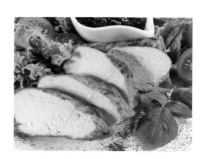
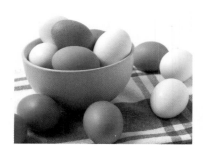
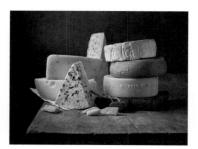

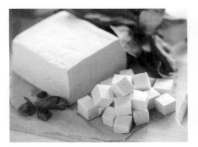
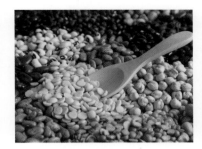
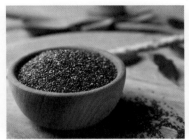
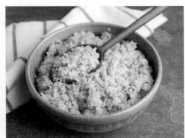

Plant-based proteins are mostly incomplete, which means in order to get all the amino acids we require, we need to eat a wide variety of these foods. This is especially important for vegetarians and vegans. Some of the best plant-based sources are:

- Soy (tofu, tempeh, and edamame).
- Legumes, such as beans, peas, chickpeas, lentils, and peanuts.
- Hemp and chia seeds.
- Quinoa.
- Seitan (a wheat-based meat alternative).

By focusing on eating good-quality, lean protein, we can not only help our waistlines, but enhance our chances of staying fit and well in later life.

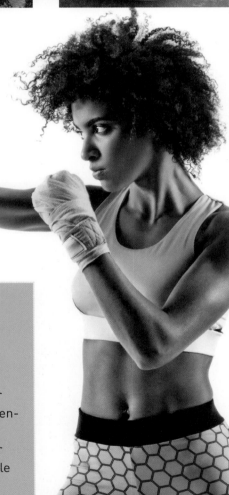

3 PROTEIN HEROES

- **Turkey** is an excellent source of lean animal protein that is healthy and affordable. Turkey mince is particularly good for making a lighter Bolognese sauce, or you can make healthy meatballs by mixing some of it with chopped herbs, a whisked egg, and fresh breadcrumbs, then pan-frying until golden.
- **Black beans** are protein-packed and full of antioxidant anthocyanins, which give them their beautiful color. Use in place of beef for a brilliant plant-based chilli, or try making some gluten-free black bean brownies for a protein-rich, tasty, power snack.
- **Quinoa** is one of the few complete plant proteins. It can be used as an alternative to rice, or you can make quinoa porridge by gently simmering with milk, vanilla extract, and some maple syrup for around 20 minutes.

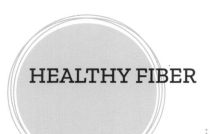

HEALTHY FIBER

Fiber is a form of carbohydrate that the body can't digest, which, as well as keeping our bowels healthy and our energy levels up, plays an important role in weight management by regulating our appetite.

Fiber makes us feel fuller for longer by delaying the emptying of food from the stomach. It also slows the absorption of glucose into the bloodstream, which prevents the hunger pangs that accompany a drop in blood sugar levels. So how much fiber do we need to eat, and which foods are fiber-rich? The recommended average intake for adults is 30 g (1 oz) per day, however, according to a recent report by the World Health Organization, only around 9 percent of adults in the UK are getting enough. One problem is that it can be difficult to visualize what 30 g (1 oz) of fiber looks like when it comes to the food on our plate, so here are a few easy ways to fill up on fiber:

WHOLEGRAIN

For breakfast, wholegrain cereals are a great choice, but be careful that they don't contain lots of sugar. An oat-based muesli contains about 5 g (⅛ oz) of fiber per 45 g (1½ oz) serving. Wholegrain bread is another easy fiber hit, containing 2–3 g (¹⁄₁₆–¹⁄₁₀ oz) per slice.

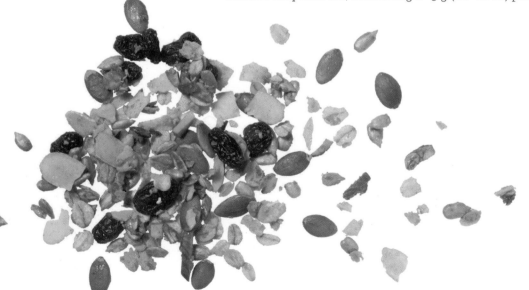

FRUIT

There are lots of fiber-rich fruits, but raspberries are top of the class with 7 g per 100 g (¼ oz per 3¾ oz). Bananas, apples, and oranges are also good.

NUTS

A snack-size portion of nuts (30 g/1 oz) contains between 2–4 g (¹⁄₁₆–⅛ oz) of fiber, with almonds, pistachios, and hazelnuts containing the most.

BAKED POTATOES

If you eat the skin as well, a medium-sized potato will give you around 4 g (⅛ oz) of fiber, which is great.

WHOLE WHEAT PASTA

A 75 g (3 oz) serving of cooked, whole wheat pasta contains 8 g (¼ oz) of fiber. This is a really easy way to get more fiber into children's diets.

PULSES

Beans, peas and lentils are all excellent sources of fiber. Half a can of baked beans contains more than 7 g (¼ oz) of fiber, an 80 g (2¾ oz) serving of frozen peas has 5 g (⅛ oz), and 100 g (¼ oz) of cooked lentils has 8 g (¼ oz) of fiber.

One final important point: Be sure to drink plenty of water throughout your day. Fiber absorbs water, so it's important to stay hydrated to enable it to do its good work in the gut and prevent constipation.

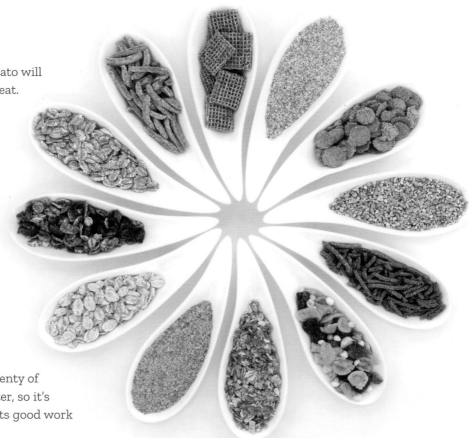

FIBER-RICH MUESLI RECIPE

Many shop-bought mueslis are high in sugar, so try making this fiber-packed version instead. Serve with the milk of your choice and top with chopped banana, grated apple, or fresh raspberries for even more fabulous fiber.

- 140 g (4¾ oz) rolled oats
- 70 g (2¾oz) wheat bran
- 58 g (2 oz) raw almonds
- 70 g (2½ oz) sliced raw mixed seeds (chia, flax, sunflower, pumpkin)
- 88 g (3 oz) raisins

Mix all the ingredients together, and store in an airtight container.

HOW TO GET A HEALTHY HEART

As well as the staples listed opposite, there are a few foods and drinks that you might be surprised to discover are good for your heart.

CHOC-A-BLOCK

Researchers at King's College London found that flavanols in cocoa could be good for your heart, as they support blood flow and improve the elasticity of arteries. Cocoa also contains magnesium, a mineral that helps you relax. Go for a bar of 70 percent dark chocolate.

PUT THE KETTLE ON

Your morning cuppa could be doing more for you than you think... Research has found that drinking four cups of tea daily may reduce the risk of high blood pressure. The effect is thought to be due to caledonites, natural compounds which stimulate the production of nitric oxide, a free radical that helps to widen blood vessels. Black and green teas have been found to be most effective.

THE CHERRY ON TOP

Did you know that cherries have been found to have heart-protective properties? Research from Northumbria University showed that cherry juice could reduce high blood pressure in a comparable way to blood pressure medication, reducing the risk of stroke and coronary heart disease.

DID YOU KNOW?
40%... that's how much you could be cutting your risk of a heart attack by eating chilli peppers four times a week! The anti-inflammatory ingredient capsaicin is thought to be behind the benefit.

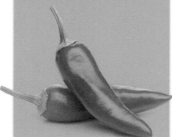

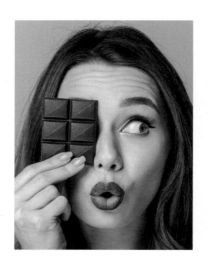
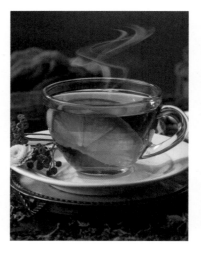
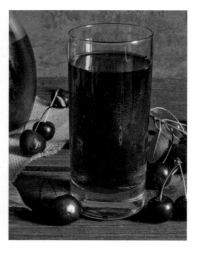

FOODS FOR A HEALTHY HEART

Keep your ticker in good working order by adding these heart-friendly foods to your diet:

- **LEAFY GREENS** contain antioxidants which help your arteries release nitric oxide, opening them up and reducing blood pressure.

- **RED AND PURPLE FOODS** such as apples, peppers, strawberries, berries, beetroot, watermelon, radishes, pomegranates, and tomatoes contain polyphenols—antioxidants that are beneficial for vascular and heart health.

- **GLOBE ARTICHOKES** inhibit the manufacture of cholesterol, as well as encouraging its breakdown and reducing its absorption in the gut. They also increase bile production and flow, thereby helping you to process fats.

- **OILY FISH** such as wild salmon, mackerel, herring, trout, and sardines are all rich in protective omega-3 fatty acids, which have an anti-inflammatory effect.

- **FLAXSEEDS/LINSEEDS** contain omega-3 fatty acids and fiber.

- **WALNUTS** contain omega-3 fatty acids.

- **OATS** are packed with fiber. They keep blood sugar levels stable and contain beta glucan, which lowers cholesterol.

- **RED WINE** contains resveratrol, a powerful antioxidant—just one glass is sufficient!

EAT TO BEAT STRESS

We've all been there—you've had a stressful day and out comes the wine and chocolate. But this might not be the best idea for your body. Let's have a look at how stress affects us, and then we'll suggest some top stress-busting foods.

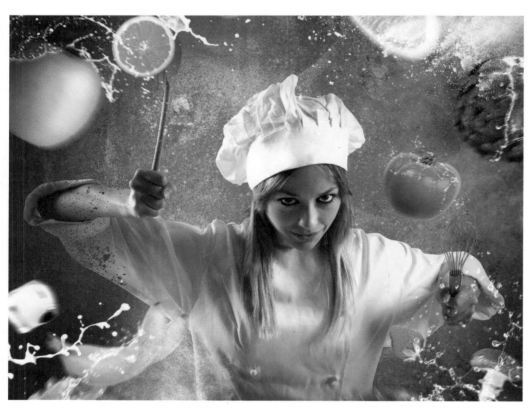

EFFECTS OF STRESS

When you are under stress, your stress hormones—including cortisol—prepare the body for a fight-or-flight response by flooding it with glucose. While this will give you a short burst of energy, when cortisol levels become elevated, over time imbalances can result. Chronic stress can lead to excess glucose, raised blood sugar levels, raised insulin, and insulin resistance. When this happens, your cells are not able to use the glucose efficiently and so it's stored as body fat. As your cells are crying out for energy, you will not only feel fatigued, but your body sends hunger signals to the brain, influencing hormones linked to appetite and cravings. This explains why we often eat when under stress. Research has also shown that stress can lead to a preference for comfort foods—typically those that are high in fat and sugar—which only aggravates the problem.

Ongoing stress can deplete many vitamins and minerals in the body, so making the right food choices is particularly important. The adrenal glands, which produce our stress hormones, require sufficient protein (particularly the amino acid tyrosine) and key nutrients such as vitamin C, B vitamins (especially Pantothenic acid B5), magnesium, zinc, and omega-3 fats. By optimizing your intake of these nutrients, you can help improve your resilience to the stress you are facing. Certain foods and nutrients can also help curb cravings and balance your blood sugar, which is often imbalanced under stress.

STRESS-BUSTING FOODS

The next time you're feeling stressed, have a look through the list below and overleaf, and try something from here instead of making an unhealthy choice that will only make you feel worse.

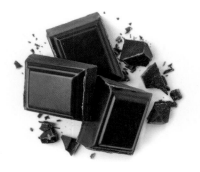

Dark chocolate

Researchers have found eating a couple of squares of dark chocolate (30 g/1 oz) can reduce stress hormones, stabilize blood glucose, and may help control cravings. This is perfect as a small treat when you need a pick me up.

Sweet potato

Provides plenty of slow-release carbohydrate to help balance blood sugar. A good source of potassium, vitamin C, and vitamin A, all of which battle stress.

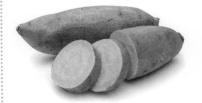

Salmon and other oily fish

Packed with anti-inflammatory omega-3 fats, shown to lower stress response. Intake of these fats has also been associated with a reduction in visceral fat. Try grilling a salmon fillet with lemon and herbs.

Apple cider vinegar

Thought to help with blood sugar balance and may improve insulin sensitivity, which in turn may support weight loss. Try drizzling it over salads or cooked vegetables.

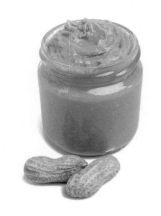

Peanut butter

High in calories but packed with protein and healthy fats to help curb appetite and cravings. Loaded with the amino acid L-tryptophan, needed for our mood-boosting neurotransmitter serotonin.

Broccoli and other greens

Low in calories but high in fiber and nutrients, including magnesium, which can help calm the mind when under stress. Fill your plate with these veggies or make a broccoli soup for a stress-busting lunch.

Grapefruit

A great source of vitamin C, which is vital for a healthy stress response. Grapefruit may also improve insulin sensitivity, which may aid weight loss. **Note:** Grapefruit can interfere with other medicines (usually making them stronger), so check with your pharmacist or doctor if you're taking any prescription medication.

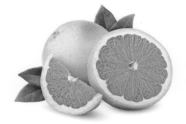

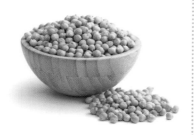

Chickpeas

Chickpeas are packed with vitamins and minerals, including magnesium, potassium, B vitamins, zinc, and selenium. The protein and fiber make them really satisfying, too. Toss a can of chickpeas in a little olive oil and paprika, and bake until crispy.

Prawns (shrimp) and other seafood

Loaded with stress-supporting nutrients, including B vitamins, zinc, and selenium. A good source of the amino acid taurine, they boost our mood through the production of dopamine. Toss prawns (shrimp) into a stir-fry.

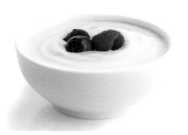

Turmeric

A potent anti-inflammatory spice shown to reduce inflammation associated with weight gain. The active component curcumin appears to also help lower anxiety and stress. Add a spoonful to smoothies.

Greek yogurt

Packed with protein to help curb cravings. Yogurt is a natural source of beneficial bacteria (probiotics), which can help reduce stress and decrease inflammation. Try a bowl of Greek yogurt with berries.

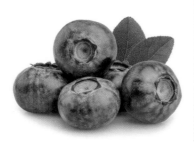

Berries

An ideal sweet treat, berries are also the perfect stress food—especially blueberries. They are loaded with flavonoid antioxidants and vitamin C to keep the body's immune system healthy. Try topping Greek yogurt with a handful of berries for a healthy stress-buster.

Turkey

Low in fat and high in protein, turkey provides plenty of the amino acid tryptophan, which is converted to serotonin to boost mood and reduce anxiety. Use turkey mince in a chilli, or shape it into burgers.

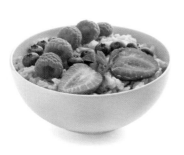

Eggs

Packed with protein and nutrients to keep you full, balance blood sugar levels and support our stress response. A good source of choline, a nutrient that is important for mood.

Oats

The combination of protein, fiber and slow-releasing carbs makes oats the ideal fuel. They provide stress-supporting nutrients including zinc, magnesium, B vitamins, iron, and manganese. Try a bowl of porridge sprinkled with cinnamon and topped with berries.

BEST STRESS-BUSTING DRINKS

Don't forget drinks as well as food! There are plenty of delicious liquids that are good for stress relief.

COCONUT WATER
• Helps to replenish vital electrolytes (potassium, sodium, and magnesium), which are often depleted when we're under stress.

MATCHA GREEN TEA
• Contains antioxidants such as epigallocatechin gallate, which has been scientifically shown to boost metabolism.

MISO SOUP
• Cravings for salt are common under stress, as the adrenal glands are involved in balancing sodium levels. Miso soup is a low-calorie warming way to satisfy your salt cravings.

TOMATO JUICE
• Provides a valuable source of vitamin C which is essential for adrenal health, and potassium which is often low when we are under stress.

CHAMOMILE TEA
• A medicinal herb used as a natural stress reducer. It has been shown to promote restful sleep and reduce the symptoms of anxiety.

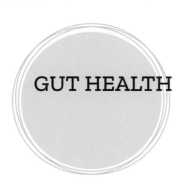

GUT HEALTH

Did you know that you have more bacteria inside your body than cells? Most of these are good for you—they help you to digest food, for example. Certain foods, because of how they are prepared, can actually boost the good bacteria, yeasts, and fungi that live inside our gut.

Below: When it comes to gut bacteria, it's a case of "the more, the merrier"—a diverse range of bacteria is best. Your "good" bacteria also keep your "bad" bacteria in check, which helps with conditions such as Crohn's disease, ulcerative colitis, and irritable bowel syndrome (IBS).

If you're feeling particularly stressed or anxious, there's a good chance what you've eaten has exacerbated or even created those uncomfortable feelings. That's because your digestive system is incredibly sensitive and comprises a whole microbiome of good bacteria. These bacteria have been found to influence weight, heart health, immunity, and levels of inflammation in your body, and now it's becoming more apparent that they also impact your mental wellbeing. "On a basic level, we've always known the gut and brain are linked—if you feel nervous, you tend to feel it in your stomach," says registered dietician Laura Clark (lecnutrition.co.uk). "But what we're now understanding is that the types of good bacteria you have, and [their] numbers, can influence the way your brain is able to cope with certain conditions." And this includes stress, anxiety, and depression. As a result, scientists have deemed our stomachs a "second brain" and, over the past few years, research has emerged revealing just how interconnected the gut and brain are. So, can the food you eat help improve your mental wellbeing?

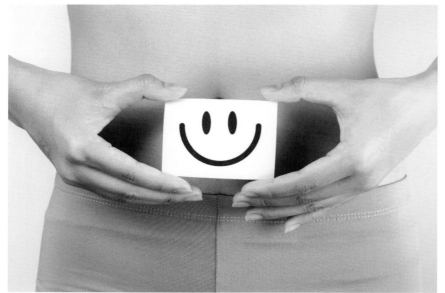

FIBER AND FERMENTED FOODS
Most of us don't get enough fiber per day—we need at least 30 g (1 oz). Fiber feeds your gut bugs and also increases the bulk and softness of your poo, which helps keep you regular. Another type of food shown to boost good gut bacteria and thereby reduce stress is fermented food, according to a scientific paper by US and Canadian researchers. "Foods such as miso, kefir, sauerkraut, and kimchi can support optimal levels of good bacteria, plus the process of fermenting the food optimises its nutrient content," says Catherine Arnold (catherinearnoldnutrition.com).

Try including some of the foods on the page opposite to support your gut and the microbes that keep you well.

Fiber

Load up on fruit and veg in their whole forms, including skins where edible. Nuts and seeds and legumes are also great. Start off slow, with an extra portion of fiber a day, and then gradually increase.

Sauerkraut

Unfermented sauerkraut is teaming with bacteria—of the good kind! The live nature of ferments means it takes some time to get used to, so start out with small amounts of sauerkraut—a teaspoon per meal—to get used to it, and see how you find it.

Kimchi

This originates from Korea, dating back more than 3,000 years, where salt was used as a method of preserving vegetables during the cold winter months. It typically contains cabbage and flavorings such as garlic, ginger, and chilli peppers. Like sauerkraut, it contains live bacteria. Start slow and build up. It's really nice with hummus.

Kombucha

A refreshing tonic of kombucha is made using live cultures referred to as "grains" or a "SCOBY" ("symbiotic culture of bacteria and yeast".) The cultures feed off the sugar in the ferments, transforming to a small amount of alcohol, acetic acid, and carbon monoxide while the microbes multiply. It is a great alternative to fizzy preservative-laden drinks.

Kefir

This fermented drink is usually made with dairy milk, but you can get it made with non-dairy milk alternatives or even water. Kefir grains are added to milk and water and ferment either sugar that is naturally present or added sugar (usually in water kefir), and the by-products turn it sour and slightly fizzy. It's an acquired taste but worth it for the extra microbes you'll be consuming. The kefir grains digest most of the lactose (milk sugar), making it easier to digest for a those who have trouble with lactose.

Sourdough

A traditional sourdough is a live culture of flour and water, referred to as a "mother" or "starter," containing a blend of *Lactobacillus* bacteria and yeast. These produce beneficial by-products that look after your gut. The minerals iron, magnesium, and zinc are also made more available by the fermentation process. A sourdough starter can be kept for ages with minimal maintenance, ready for whenever you want to bake.

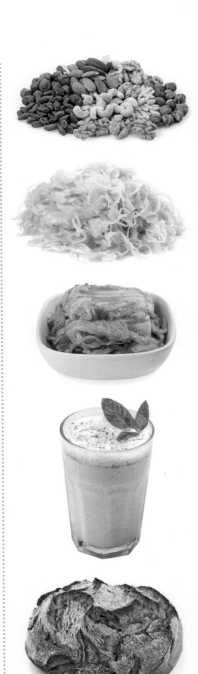

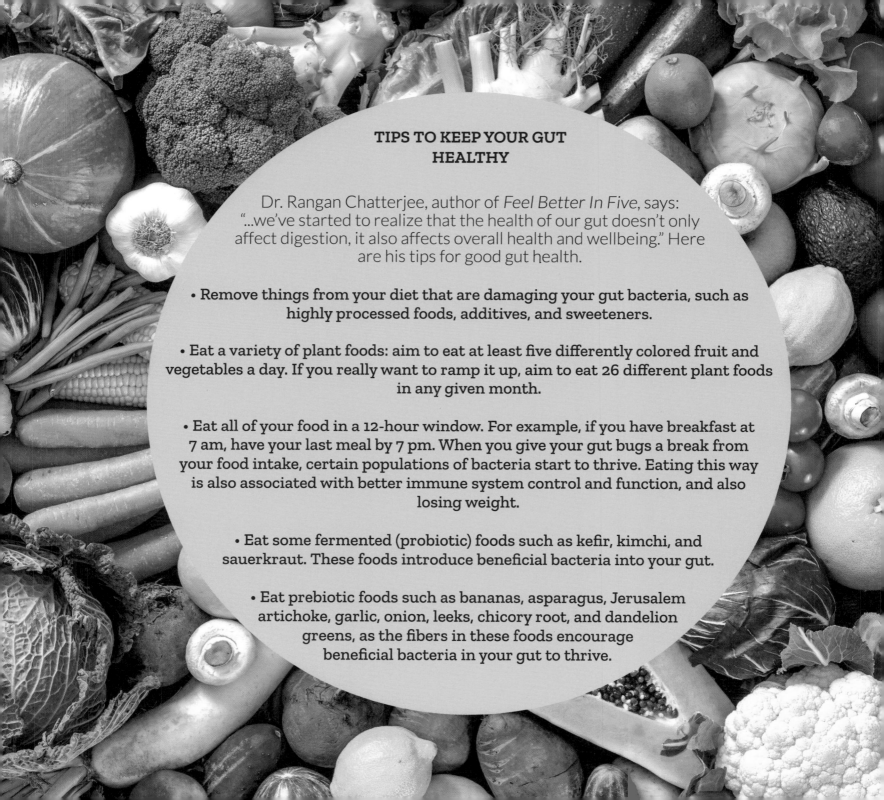

TIPS TO KEEP YOUR GUT HEALTHY

Dr. Rangan Chatterjee, author of *Feel Better In Five*, says: "...we've started to realize that the health of our gut doesn't only affect digestion, it also affects overall health and wellbeing." Here are his tips for good gut health.

• Remove things from your diet that are damaging your gut bacteria, such as highly processed foods, additives, and sweeteners.

• Eat a variety of plant foods: aim to eat at least five differently colored fruit and vegetables a day. If you really want to ramp it up, aim to eat 26 different plant foods in any given month.

• Eat all of your food in a 12-hour window. For example, if you have breakfast at 7 am, have your last meal by 7 pm. When you give your gut bugs a break from your food intake, certain populations of bacteria start to thrive. Eating this way is also associated with better immune system control and function, and also losing weight.

• Eat some fermented (probiotic) foods such as kefir, kimchi, and sauerkraut. These foods introduce beneficial bacteria into your gut.

• Eat prebiotic foods such as bananas, asparagus, Jerusalem artichoke, garlic, onion, leeks, chicory root, and dandelion greens, as the fibers in these foods encourage beneficial bacteria in your gut to thrive.

HEALTHY GUT, HEALTHY BRAIN

The latest scientific research suggests that Parkinson's disease may originate in the gut. If so, could treating the microbiome be a way to prevent and/or manage the condition?

Think of Parkinson's disease and you might naturally consider it a purely brain-based condition. But latest studies suggest that the gut may have an important role to play. "We are increasingly finding out more about the gut microbiome in relation to health and disease," says Professor Glenn Gibson, head of Food Microbial Sciences at the University of Reading. "The connection that the gut could be involved in migraine and schizophrenia was first made in the 1800s. This was not taken seriously at the time. But we now know that the gut microbiome is central to many disorders. These include cognitive issues, anxiety, depression, migraines, autism, dementia, and now also Parkinson's disease." Parkinson's disease is a progressive neurological condition. The three main symptoms are tremor, muscle stiffness, and slowness of movement. Other symptoms may include tiredness, pain, depression, and mood changes. Latest figures from Parkinson's UK (parkinsons.org.uk) estimate that around 145,000 people (that's one adult in 350) are diagnosed with it and it mostly affects people over 50, but younger people get it, too. People with Parkinson's don't produce enough of the hormone dopamine, the pleasure hormone. There is no current cure, and the main treatment is medication to restore levels of dopamine. This can have side effects, though (involuntary movements and impulsive, compulsive behavior). Other treatments include deep brain stimulation, and physical therapies such as physiotherapy, speech, and occupational therapy.

EAT YOURSELF HAPPY

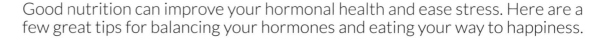

Good nutrition can improve your hormonal health and ease stress. Here are a few great tips for balancing your hormones and eating your way to happiness.

To stay healthy, you need to keep your hormones in balance. "For your hormones to function well, you need to eat a healthy, varied diet to ensure you get all the essential nutrients," says nutritional therapist Angelique Panagos. "This means healthy fats (e.g. avocados, nuts, seeds, olive oil), carbohydrates (e.g. vegetables and whole grains) and proteins (e.g. organic meat, fish, lentils, chickpeas). Good gut health is also crucial as if your gut isn't working, you won't absorb nutrients properly." Just as eating a nutritious diet will help to support hormones, the reverse is also true. "Dietary stresses are a major contributor to hormonal imbalance," says Angelique. "This can be consuming the wrong foods, over-eating or skipping meals—things we all do occasionally without realizing the effect on hormones. Not getting enough healthy fats, for example, reduces your ability to makes hormones and also deprives you of essential, fat-soluble nutrients such as vitamins A, D, E, and K. Here are some good food and behavioral practices:

- **EAT WHOLE FOOD, NOT PROCESSED FOOD.** Dump the junk. Processed foods are devoid of nutrients.
- **EAT THE RIGHT CARBS... NOT NO CARBS.** Go for fibrous whole grains and vegetables. These are high in nutrients and fiber, essential for healthy waste elimination. Avoid refined white carbs (such as bread, pasta, and white rice), and say no to added sugar or artificial sweeteners.
- **EAT GOOD FATS DAILY.** Go for olive oil, avocado, nuts, and seeds. Fat does not make you fat; sugar does. Eating the right fats builds hormones and keeps your cells and skin supple. Healthy fats also have a beneficial, anti-inflammatory effect on your body.
- **EAT REGULARLY AND INCLUDE SOME PROTEIN IN EVERY MEAL.** This will help to keep your blood sugar levels balanced.
- **EAT A RAINBOW OF VEGETABLES.** The wider the variety of colors in your meals, the more vitamins and minerals you'll pack in.
- **GO ORGANIC WHERE POSSIBLE.** This reduces the toxic burden on your body and helps with your hormonal balance. Exposure to xenoestrogens, antibiotics, and hormones in animal products, chemicals, and pesticides are hormone disruptors.
- **TAKE A 30-MINUTE BREAK TO EAT IN PEACE.** This will allow you to eat consciously and slowly. If you eat while stressed, blood is diverted away from the digestive system, leading to bloating. Eating mindlessly also makes you eat more than you need.

> "If more of us valued food and cheer and song above hoarded gold, it would be a merrier world."
> J.R.R. Tolkien

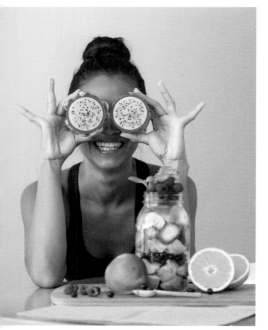

MEALS TO EASE STRESS

Try the following meal plans to balance your hormones, boost vitality and improve your gut health and mental wellbeing. Drinks could include water, peppermint tea, ginger tea, turmeric tea latte or probiotic shots.

DAY 1
Breakfast: No-added sugar live yogurt with chopped banana, 1 tbsp flaxseed, nuts/seeds.
Lunch: Slice of rye bread toast with two poached eggs, asparagus, and some spinach.
Dinner: Mixed beans with kale, organic chicken breast, broccoli, and lemon juice.
Snacks: Miso soup with nori, two squares of dark chocolate.

DAY 2
Breakfast: Banana and blueberry pancakes, with coconut yogurt.
Lunch: Greek salad with chickpeas, drizzled with olive oil.
Dinner: Grilled salmon fillet with lentils and broccoli.
Snacks: Small handful of almonds, an orange.

DAY 3
Breakfast: Spinach and mushroom omelette.
Lunch: Buckwheat noodles with cubed tofu, edamame beans, and miso dressing.
Dinner: Baked sweet potato with hummus and sweetcorn, green salad sprinkled with seeds.
Snacks: Two brown rice crackers with nut butter, handful of blackberries.

DAY 4
Breakfast: Porridge with mixed berries, 1 tbsp flaxseed and some nutans seeds.
Lunch: Quinoa, broccoli, and poached egg on a bed of kale.
Dinner: Squash and tomato curry with brown rice.
Snacks: Two squares of dark chocolate, two nectarines.

DAY 5
Breakfast: Cacao chia seed pudding.
Lunch: Green leaf salad topped with black beans, roasted (bell) peppers, and some grilled courgette (zucchini).
Dinner: Miso chicken with brown rice and kimchi.
Snacks: Small handful of pumpkin seeds, an apple.

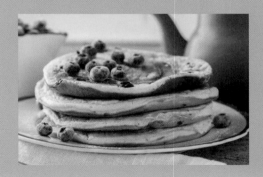
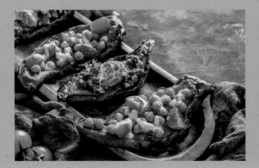
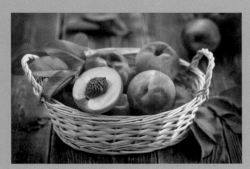

FEELING FRISKY?

Some foods are widely thought to boost libido. Here's a list of aphrodisiac foods that may put you in the mood for love...

Seafood (such as oysters, mussels, and fish) are high in zinc, phosphorus, and iodine, all vital for sexual health.

Vanilla scent has been shown in studies to have an aphrodisiac effect.

Chillies contain capsaicin, which stimulates circulation and improves sexual desire.

Sweet potato, pumpkin, and avocado support hormonal health.

Walnuts are packed with essential fatty acids that help to regulate hormone levels.

Brazil nuts are high in selenium, essential for a healthy thyroid.

Asparagus contains asparagocide, a plant hormone reputed to increase libido. It is also packed with selenium, and vitamins A and C, all important nutrients for healthy sexual function.

Figs contain beneficial vitamins and minerals, including vitamins, E and B6, manganese, calcium, and potassium.

Dates are rich in amino acids, known to increase sexual stamina.

Pomegranate helps to increase testosterone levels (one of the hormones that boosts libido) in both men and women.

Chocolate contains phenylethylamine, an amphetamine-like substance that heightens desire.

Licorice root is used in Chinese medicine to boost women's libido.

A–Z OF FOODS TO KEEP YOU YOUNG

The foods we eat lay the foundations for our health as we age, so it's a good idea to get into good habits. Here is an A–Z list of foods and supplements that will help you to live your healthiest life for a long time to come.

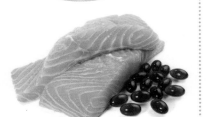

A is for ASTAXANTHIN

This naturally occurring carotenoid found in algae and fish, such as shrimp, lobster, and crab, is one of nature's most powerful antioxidants. Hailed as a hero for joint pain, it's also believed to slow cognitive decline and promote the growth of new brain cells, keeping your mind young.

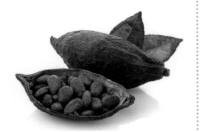

B is for BASIL

Relight your libido with the aphrodisiac herb! Basil is said to help increase blood flow throughout your body and is a great source of vitamin A, beta-carotene, magnesium, potassium, and vitamin C, which work in harmony to boost sexual desire.

C is for CACAO

It's hard to beat that feeling of contentment as you indulge in a square of dark chocolate! Raw cacao boosts serotonin and endorphins known to create feelings of happiness. Not only this, its high flavanol content also improves blood flow, resulting in better circulation and brighter skin.

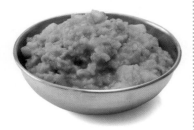

D is for DHAL

With youth-boosting benefits aplenty, we should all be tucking into this more often. It's believed that legumes, including lentils, beans, and peas, help to stabilize blood sugar, lower cholesterol, and nourish your teeth and bones, keeping them stronger and healthier for longer.

E is for EVENING PRIMROSE OIL

This skin savior hydrates, plumps, and smooths, as well as reducing skin blemishes. It's also said to help alleviate hot flushes and other menopausal symptoms.

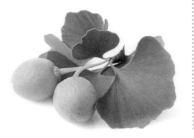

G is for GINKGO

This plucky plant contains powerful antioxidants that fight inflammation and support brain health. Nutritional therapist Alison Cullen says, "ginkgo is known to have a protective effect on serotonin sites in your brain, which leads to an increased ability to focus and recall information."

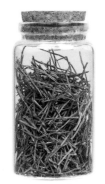

H is for HORSETAIL

Thicker, fuller tresses are a sure sign of youth. Thanks, to its high silica content, horsetail not only stimulates hair growth but also cleanses and soothes your scalp, leaving locks rejuvenated.

I is for INDIAN BLACKTAIL

Indian black salt has been used in Ayurvedic medicines and therapies for centuries. It contains less sodium than table salt, reducing water retention and bloating, while its alkaline properties help tackle excess stomach acid, preventing acid reflux.

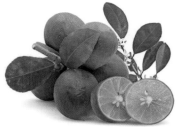

J is for JUJUBE FRUIT

Also known as red dates, jujube fruits can help calm your body and mind, helping you switch off and get plenty of beauty sleep. Not only this, their rich antioxidant and vitamin content can also help fight free radicals and bolster your immune system.

K is for KAFFIR LIME

Essential oils from kaffir lime leaves can destroy acne-causing bacteria and reduce the formation of scars and blemishes on your skin.

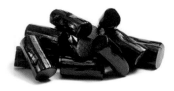

L is for LIQUORICE

Soothe heartburn with this childhood favorite. Its anti-inflammatory and immune-boosting glycyrrhizic acid content is why it works.

M is for MAGNESIUM

Lower your blood pressure with magnesium. Studies found that people with high blood pressure who started taking magnesium every day saw it drop significantly. Dark chocolate, avocado, and tofu are just a few magnesium-rich foods.

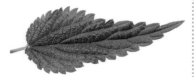

N is for NETTLE

This prickly plant has less of a sting when ingested as a warming brew or in supplement form. A natural diuretic, nettle is said to rejuvenate your liver and aid healing.

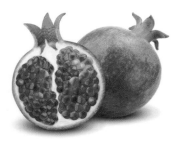

P is for POMEGRANATE

The punchy, pink pomegranate contains antioxidants that help slow the natural breakdown of DNA in your cells. Just one glass of pomegranate juice a day could be all it takes, but remember to choose one with no added sugar or it will undo all the good work.

Q is for QUERCETIN

Quercetin is a type of flavonoid antioxidant that's found in dark-colored foods, such as leafy greens, tomatoes, berries, and cherries, as well as in citrus fruits, grapes, apples, onions, parsley, sage, tea, red wine, and olive oil. It improves endurance, helping you exercise for longer.

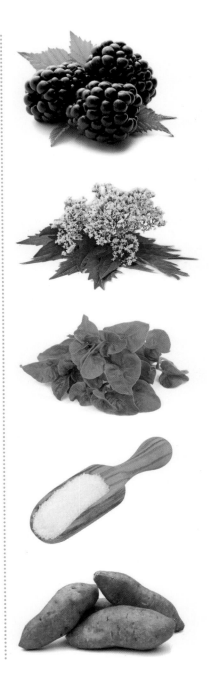

R is for ROSEMARY

This versatile herb goes with so many dishes—meat, fish, soups, and stews—and its benefits are just as numerous. Perhaps most impressive is its ability to slow brain ageing and enhance memory.

T is for TURMERIC

Curcumin, turmeric's active compound, is thought to prevent a number of age-related diseases, including heart disease and Alzheimer's.

V is for VALERIAN

Good-quality sleep is key to staying young, as your body repairs overnight. Help sleep with valerian root, which is hailed as a cure for insomnia.

W is for WATERCRESS

This peppery powerhouse contains more than 50 vitamins and minerals. It actually contains more calcium than milk, more vitamin C than an orange, and more folate than a banana. It also has high levels of phenethyl isothiocyanate (PEITC), which scientific research has found reduces DNA damage. Chew it well to maximize the benefits.

X is for XYLITOL

Still craving the sweet stuff? Try xylitol, the low-sugar alternative derived from birch and beech wood. It is believed to have antibacterial properties and is said to be good for your teeth.

Y is for YAMS

A great source of fiber, potassium, manganese, and copper, yams are thought to help stabilize estrogen (oestrogen) levels, lessening menopause symptoms. Available in most supermarkets, they make a healthy alternative to the humble potato.

Z is for ZINC

This essential mineral is a must for boosting your immune system, helping with the production of skin cells and reducing inflammation.

BENEFITS
OF BEING A LITTLE
LIGHTER

We're not talking about fitting into the skinny jeans that you wore as a teenager, but there are very real health benefits in reducing your body weight by even a small amount. Here are some of the ways in which you'll feel better:

• JOINT PROTECTION: You'll ease the pressure on your knees and other lower body joints, making you less likely to develop arthritis in later life.

• EASIER TO EXERCISE: You'll move better and find that your stamina improves.

• LESS BACK PAIN: You'll have less pressure on your spinal discs—every pound you lose equates to 16 pounds of pressure on your spine!

• LOWERED RISK OF DIABETES: You'll help stabilize your blood sugar levels and potentially lower your need for medication.

• IMPROVED HEART HEALTH AND LOWER BLOOD PRESSURE: Your heart won't have to work as hard to move blood around your body.

• REDUCED RISK OF CANCER: With less fat, you'll have lower levels of some of the hormones linked to cancer, such as estrogen (oestrogen), insulin, and androgen.

• BETTER SLEEP: You'll breathe more easily, with less sleep apnea and snoring. A better night's sleep will improve your mood and energy levels.

TWO WEEKS TO A LIGHTER YOU!

For anyone who would like to be a little lighter, the remainder of this chapter plots out a two-week plan with practical ideas for the sorts of foods—and their quantities—that will help you. Some of the recipes from the plan are included at the end of the chapter.

PROTEIN: Eat some good-quality protein with every meal to keep your blood sugar levels balanced. Protein also helps to speed up your metabolism so that you burn fat more efficiently.

VEGETABLES: The types of vegetables that grow above the ground—such as asparagus, lettuce, spinach, cabbage, cauliflower, green beans, (bell) peppers, tomatoes, aubergine (eggplant), avocado, kale, courgette (zucchini), olives, and avocado—are lower in carbs and have a lower glycaemic index compared to below-ground veggies, so won't cause your blood sugar to spike. Root vegetables are starchier and richer in natural sugars.

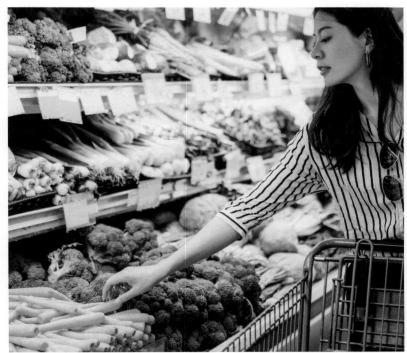

FRUIT: Eat fruit every day! If you prefer low-carb and low-glycaemic choices, go for raspberries and blackberries.

HEALTHY FATS: You'll find these in olive oil, coconut milk, nuts, seeds, oily fish, yogurt, avocados, and vegetable oils, which are sources of slow-burn energy that help to stabilize blood sugar.

DRINKS: Take mineral water, herbal teas such as green tea, fennel, ginger, dandelion, matcha, and fresh mint. It's perfectly fine to have one cup of tea or coffee per day.

THERMOGENIC SPICES: These are fat-burning spices, and include chilli, turmeric, and cayenne pepper. Studies show that these help to speed up your metabolism and increase fat burning.

GO ORGANIC: When shopping, look for good-quality, organic meat, sustainable sources of fish and seafood, and organic vegetables whenever possible.

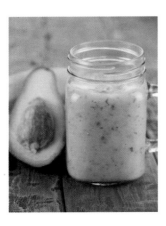

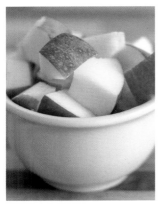

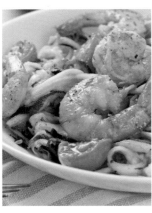

WEEK ONE

MONDAY
BREAKFAST: Avocado Breakfast Booster (SEE RECIPE, page 128).
MID-MORNING SNACK: 1 sliced apple with 2 tsp almond butter.
LUNCH: Serve 1 poached egg with 95 g (3⅓ oz) canned sardines and spinach. Season with paprika, chilli, and tamari.
MID-AFTERNOON SNACK: 1 tbsp sunflower seeds and two squares of dark chocolate (70 percent cacao).
DINNER: Stir-fry tofu, pak choi, mangetouts (sugar peas), spring onions (scallions), and bean sprouts with garlic, fresh ginger, and soy sauce. Sprinkle with 20 g (⅔ oz) toasted cashews.

TUESDAY
BREAKFAST: Coconut Quinoa Porridge (SEE RECIPE, page 128).
MID-MORNING SNACK: 12 almonds.
LUNCH: Serve 1 smoked mackerel fillet with steamed tenderstem broccoli and green beans.
MID-AFTERNOON SNACK: 6 brazil nuts.
DINNER: Top courgetti (zucchini noodles) with prawns (shrimp). Drizzle with olive oil and season with cayenne and fresh chillies.

WEDNESDAY
BREAKFAST: Scramble 2 eggs with 50 g (1⅔ oz) smoked salmon and parsley.
MID-MORNING SNACK: 1 sliced apple with 2 tbsp cashew butter.
LUNCH: Spiralize 1 large courgette (zucchini). Heat in a pan with dollop of basil pesto. Top with 20 g (⅔ oz) toasted pine nuts. Garnish with fresh basil leaves.
MID-AFTERNOON SNACK: 4 walnut halves.
DINNER: Stir-fry 100 g (3½ oz) chicken strips with green chillies, green beans, pak choi, spring onions (scallions), ½ tbsp Thai fish sauce, and some coconut milk.

THURSDAY
BREAKFAST: Blend a handful of blueberries, 200 ml (scant 1 cup) unsweetened coconut milk, handful baby spinach, 1 tsp flaxseed, 1 tsp sunflower seeds, and 1 scoop of plant-based protein powder.
MID-MORNING SNACK: 5 brazil nuts.
LUNCH: Mix some leaves with 6 olives, 4 cherry tomatoes, chopped red onion, and a little feta cheese.
MID-AFTERNOON SNACK: 125 g (4¼ oz) pot of coconut yogurt.
DINNER: Grill 1 salmon fillet, drizzle with olive oil and lemon. Serve with spinach.

FRIDAY
BREAKFAST: Mix 2 tbsp almond butter with 2 tsp mixed seeds and goji berries. Use apple wedges to dip into the mixture.
MID-MORNING SNACK: 1–2 tbsp pumpkin seeds.
LUNCH: Top 100 g (3½ oz) tinned mackerel with baby spinach, chopped red onion, 2 spring onions (scallions) and a boiled egg.
MID-AFTERNOON SNACK: Spiralized apple with 2 tbsp almond butter.
DINNER: Cauliflower Curry (SEE RECIPE, page 128).

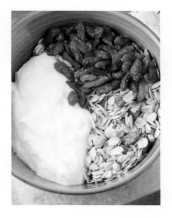

SATURDAY
BREAKFAST: Make a 2-egg omelette with 50 g (1⅔ oz) salmon. Serve with 30 g (1 oz) asparagus.
MID-MORNING SNACK: 1 Granny Smith apple with 3 walnuts.
LUNCH: Grill 2 slices (25 g/scant 1 oz) halloumi and a Portobello mushroom. Serve with a green salad.
MID-AFTERNOON SNACK: 1 tbsp mixed seeds.
DINNER: Season 100 g (3½ oz) cubed chicken with paprika. Place on skewer with chopped (bell) peppers, aubergine (egglant), and courgette (zucchini), and grill.

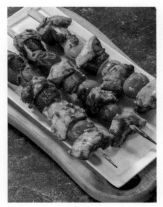

SUNDAY
BREAKFAST: Serve 125 g (4¼ oz) coconut yogurt with 20 g (⅔ oz) nuts and seeds.
MID-MORNING SNACK: 1 boiled egg.
LUNCH: Serve ½ tin sardines in tomato sauce on mashed avocado, with black pepper and lime juice.
MID-AFTERNOON SNACK: 1 cup matcha green tea with 3 squares of dark chocolate.
DINNER: Mix 200 ml (scant 1 cup) coconut milk with 1–2 tsp Thai green curry paste in a pan. Add courgette (zucchini), broccoli florets, mangetouts (sugar peas), and green (bell) pepper. Simmer until done. Add 100 g (3½ oz) cooked chicken, tofu, or prawns (shrimp).

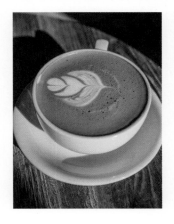

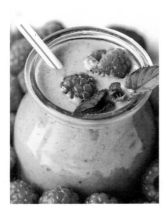

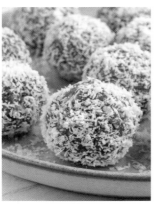

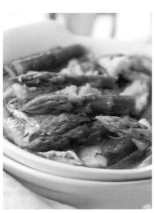

WEEK TWO

MONDAY
BREAKFAST: Berry Blast (SEE RECIPE, page 129).
MID-MORNING SNACK: Green tea with 1 bsp sunflower seeds.
LUNCH: Mixed salad with mozzarella and 100 g (3½ oz) grilled turkey breast.
MID-AFTERNOON SNACK: 1 boiled egg.
DINNER: Grill 1 lamb chop, seasoned with rosemary. Serve with cauliflower rice and broccoli.

TUESDAY
BREAKFAST: Poached egg on smashed avocado with chilli flakes.
MID-MORNING SNACK: Small can of tuna.
LUNCH: Add some chicken, cauliflower, cabbage, ginger, turmeric, black pepper, Himalayan sea salt, and herbs to 200 ml (scant 1 cup) water to make soup. Simmer until the chicken is cooked through.
MID-AFTERNOON SNACK: 1 Granny Smith apple with 2 tbsp almond butter.
DINNER: Grill 1 sea bass fillet. Serve with roasted, chopped courgette (zucchini), aubergine (eggplant), tomatoes, and red (bell) peppers.

WEDNESDAY
BREAKFAST: Soak 2 tbsp chia seeds, 2 tbsp coconut yogurt and 20 chopped nuts (walnuts, hazelnuts) in 200 ml (scant 1 cup) almond milk overnight.
MID-MORNING SNACK: Sardines.
LUNCH: Chop a medium aubergine (eggplant) into slices, drizzle with olive oil and grill. Serve with 20 g (⅔ oz) goat's cheese and a small salad.
MID-AFTERNOON SNACK: 2 Coconut and Peanut Butter Balls (SEE RECIPE, page 129).
DINNER: Serve 1 grilled chicken breast with courgetti (zucchini noodles).

THURSDAY
BREAKFAST: Serve 2 vegetarian sausages with grilled tomato.
MID-MORNING SNACK: 125 g (4¼ oz) Greek-style yogurt with almond slivers.
LUNCH: Mix 2 eggs, 20 g (⅔ oz) grated cheese and cooked asparagus. Heat in a pan, then bake.
MID-AFTERNOON SNACK: 8 macadamia nuts.
DINNER: Mix 200 ml (scant 1 cup) coconut milk with 1–2 tsp red curry paste in a pan. Add courgette (zucchini), broccoli florets, mangetouts (sugar peas), and red (bell) pepper. Simmer until done. Add 100 g (3½ oz) cooked chicken, tofu, or prawns (shrimp).

FRIDAY
BREAKFAST: Top 1 small slice of grain-free bread (made without seeds, available in health stores) with cashew nut butter.
MID-MORNING SNACK: 10 almonds or cashews (unsalted).
LUNCH: Mix 40 g (1¼ oz) cooked quinoa with baby spinach, tomatoes, and 100 g (3½ oz) grilled chicken.
MID-AFTERNOON SNACK: 1 boiled egg.
DINNER: Serve 1 grilled cod fillet with green vegetables.

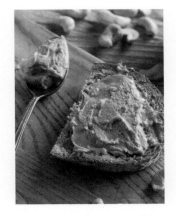

SATURDAY
BREAKFAST: Blend a handful of blueberries, 200 ml (scant 1 cup) coconut milk and a handful of kale with 1 tsp flaxseed and 1 tsp sesame seeds. Add 1 scoop of plant-based protein powder.
MID-MORNING SNACK: Half an avocado.
LUNCH: Drizzle 6 king prawns (jumbo shrimp) with lemon juice. Thread them onto skewers with some chopped red (bell) peppers, courgette (zucchini) pieces, and mushrooms. Grill until everything is cooked through.
MID-AFTERNOON SNACK: Turmeric latte with 6 almonds. Add 1 tsp turmeric and a pinch of black pepper to almond milk. Sprinkle with cinnamon.
DINNER: Cook 100 g (3½ oz) chicken thighs with sautéed onions, courgettes (zucchini), aubergines (eggplant) and (bell) peppers, garlic, ginger, turmeric, black pepper, oregano, water, and vegetable stock.

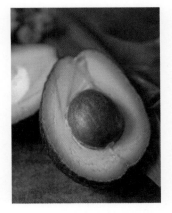

SUNDAY
BREAKFAST: Crumble 25 g (1 oz) goat's cheese on a grilled Portobello mushroom. Sprinkle with pine nuts.
MID-MORNING SNACK: 1 boiled egg.
LUNCH: Tofu Green Beans with Quinoa (SEE RECIPE, page 129)
MID-AFTERNOON SNACK: 125 g (4¼ oz) Greek-style yogurt.
DINNER: Top 1 grilled trout fillet with chopped, toasted almonds. Serve with sweetheart cabbage and asparagus.

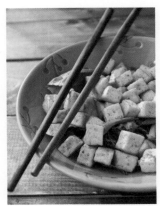

RECIPES

AVOCADO BREAKFAST BOOSTER

Serves 1

Start the day with this power-packed smoothie.

- 1 avocado
- A handful of baby spinach
- 1 scoop of hemp protein powder
- 200 ml (scant 1 cup) unsweetened coconut milk
- 1 tsp flaxseed

Place all the ingredients in a food blender and process until smooth.

COCONUT QUINOA PORRIDGE

Serves 1

Combine quinoa with three types of coconut to make this nutritious, creamy breakfast.

- 1 tbsp chia seeds
- 230 ml (1 cup) unsweetened coconut milk
- 40 g (1¼ oz) quinoa, uncooked
- A pinch of nutmeg
- 2 tbsp coconut yogurt
- 1 tbsp coconut flakes
- A handful of small berries

1. Soak the chia seeds in 30 ml (2 tbsp) coconut milk overnight.
2. Next morning, rinse the quinoa in running water. Place in a pan with the coconut milk and nutmeg. Simmer on a low heat for 15 minutes, or until the quinoa is tender.
3. Add the chia seed mix and simmer for 1 minute.
4. Stir in the coconut yogurt. Top with the coconut flakes and berries.

CAULIFLOWER CURRY

Serves 1

This tasty cauliflower curry is infused with healthy, warming spices.

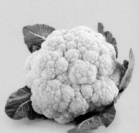

- 1 tbsp sesame oil
- 1 tbsp yellow curry paste
- ½ clove finely chopped garlic
- 150 ml (5 oz) tinned coconut milk
- 150 ml (5 oz) vegetable broth
- A handful of cauliflower florets
- 1 cm (⅓ in) slice of ginger
- ½ red (bell) pepper, seeded and cut into strips
- 20 g (⅔ oz) organic bamboo sprouts
- 50 g (1 ⅔ oz) button mushrooms, sliced
- 1 tbsp tamari
- 75 g (2 ⅔ oz) organic chicken, cooked and cut into chunks
- ½ small cauliflower (for cauliflower rice)
- 15 g (½oz) unsalted cashew nuts

1. In a wok, heat the sesame oil over medium heat until hot. Add the curry paste and garlic. Stir and cook for 1 minute.
2. Stir in the coconut milk and vegetable broth. Reduce the heat to simmer. Add the cauliflower florets and cook for 10 minutes.
3. Add the ginger, pepper strips, and bamboo sprouts. Cook until tender.
4. Add the mushrooms, tamari, and cooked chicken chunks. Simmer for another 15 minutes.
5. Blitz the cauliflower in a blender to make cauliflower rice. Steam in a covered pan for 5 minutes to cook.
6. Serve the curry with cauliflower rice and garnish with cashew nuts.

BERRY BLAST

Serves 1

Make this berry smoothie in minutes to turbo-charge your energy all day.

- 20 g (⅔ oz) strawberries
- 20 g (⅔ oz) raspberries
- 1 tsp flaxseed
- 200 ml (scant 1 cup) unsweetened coconut milk
- 1 scoop of plant-based protein powder

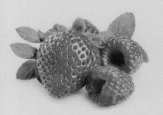

Place all the ingredients in a food blender and process until smooth.

COCONUT PEANUT BUTTER BALLS

Makes 5 servings (5 balls)

These protein-packed treats make the perfect mid-afternoon snack.

- 1 tbsp smooth peanut butter
- 1 tsp unsweetened cocoa powder
- ½ tsp stevia
- 1 tsp almond flour
- 20 g (⅔ oz) unsweetened, desiccated coconut

1. In a bowl, mix the peanut butter, cocoa powder, stevia, and almond flour.
2. Freeze for 1 hour.
3. Using an ice cream scoop, scoop out five balls and drop into the desiccated coconut so that it covers each ball.
4. Refrigerate the balls overnight, to firm them up.
5. Keep them in the fridge where they will stay fresh for 2–3 days.

TOFU GREEN BEANS WITH QUINOA

Serves 1

The spicy green curry paste gives green beans, tofu, and quinoa a delicious kick.

- 40 g (1¼ oz) red quinoa, uncooked
- 200 ml (scant 1 cup) unsweetened coconut milk
- 5–6 tsp green curry paste
- 30 g (1 oz) green beans, rinsed and trimmed
- 100 g (3½ oz) tofu, cut into cubes
- 20 g (⅔ oz) unsalted cashew nuts
- A handful of spinach leaves
- Salt

1. Rinse the quinoa under cold running water.
2. Place in a pan with double the amount of water. Add a dash of salt, to taste. Place on a medium heat and bring to the boil.
3. Reduce the heat and simmer for 10–15 minutes, until the quinoa is tender and fluffy. Leave for 1 minute.
4. While the quinoa is cooking, mix the coconut milk with the green curry paste in a separate pan. Add the green beans and simmer for 10 minutes until tender.
5. Add the tofu cubes and cashews, and simmer for 1–2 minutes.
6. Put the spinach leaves in a small pan with a dash of olive oil and heat for 1 minute, until wilted.
7. Place the quinoa in a bowl and top with the green beans and tofu.
8. Garnish with the spinach.

AND FINALLY...

Eat healthily with lots of vegetables and no processed, junk or fast foods. Once you're no longer trying to lose weight, you can re-introduce some more carby foods such as potatoes, sweet potatoes, rice, and whole wheat bread. Whatever your food plan, always try to eat moderate, healthy portions.

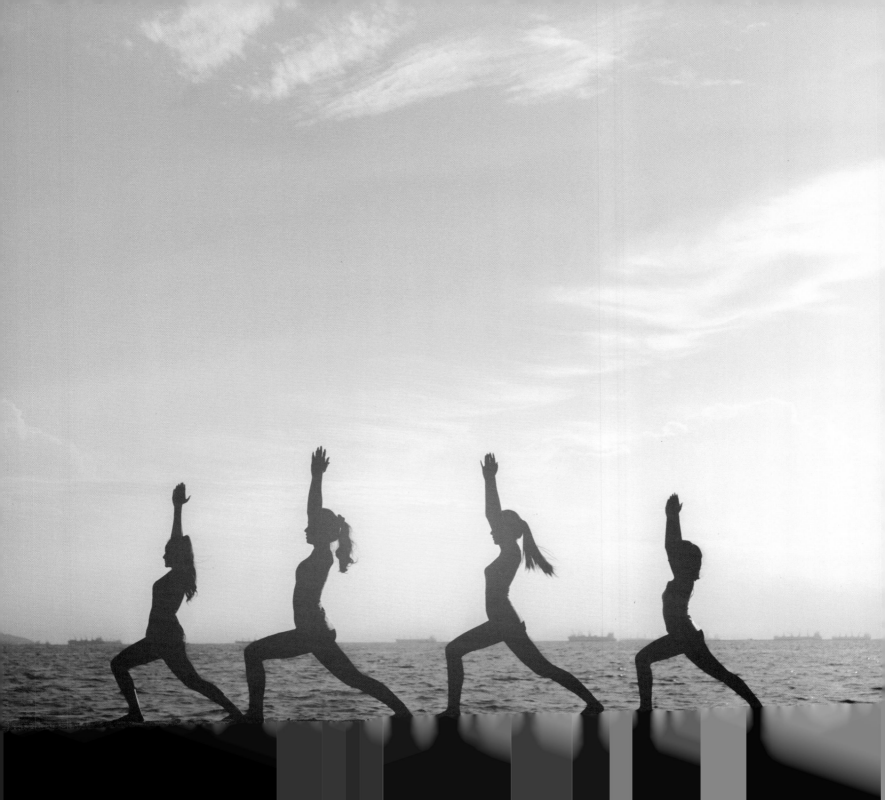

4

MOVE YOUR BODY

Human beings are meant to move—we have evolved to be physically active, with movement not only being important for almost every system in our body, but also important for cultural and social reasons. Activity makes us feel good and lowers our risk of all manner of diseases and health problems, and it's been shown that even a few minutes of exercise has incredible transformative powers, both physically and mentally.

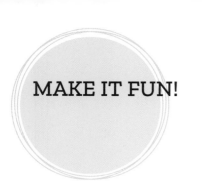

MAKE IT FUN!

The best way to stick to a regular exercise routine is to find something you enjoy. Here's how to find what works for you.

"I should really do some exercise. I feel good afterwards, but when I'm exercising it's such a chore." You've probably heard reluctant exercisers use these phrases before. Read them again and you'll see one thing. They both describe negative relationships with exercise. And this is the problem. We all know that we need to be physically active to be healthy, but many of us simply don't enjoy exercise. In our view, the only way to start and stick to an exercise routine in the long term is to find something you enjoy—something that is your personal preference, not what you think you should do or what your friends recommend. You may not love it, you may have days when you feel like skipping a workout because you're tired, but, ideally, it shouldn't be a chore. It's common to hear people say they 'should' take up running because they've heard it burns lots of calories. Others will say they "should" go to the gym because their friend went and lost a lot of weight. But any sentence that contains the word "should" when it comes to exercise is likely to be negative. If you want to stick to a regular exercise routine, it has to be something you can enjoy to a reasonable level. Willpower will work in the short term, but it will only last so long.

BE IMAGINATIVE
Put past experiences to one side and think about what appeals to you now. If you don't like getting hot and sweaty, then strength training might be better than high-intensity exercise classes. If you prefer to

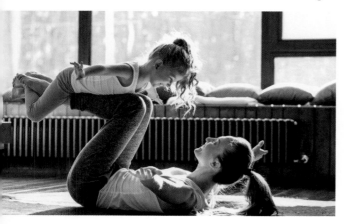

embrace the mental and spiritual benefits of exercise, then yoga might be for you. If you like the idea of being on your own and not interacting with others while you exercise, swimming or running could be ideal. Both can be solitary pursuits and offer you that invaluable "me time" and a chance to clear your head and get rid of the stresses of everyday life. Many people often ask fitness experts what the best form of exercise is for health or weight loss. Some experts will give specific answers, describing high-intensity exercise like spinning or running as the best for weight loss. Our answer would be to find the exercise that you enjoy, because that way you'll keep doing it. Running only works if you do it regularly. Exercise classes only work if you are motivated to turn up and participate at least three times per week.

It pays to be imaginative when thinking about what sort of exercise you'd like to do. Have a look at the ideas on the page opposite for inspiration.

THINK OUTSIDE THE BOX

As well as the usual exercises of walking, running, cycling, swimming, going to the gym, and playing sports, there are plenty of alternative ways to make exercise fun. If you think outside the box, perhaps some of the following might excite you, and you may even forget you are exercising!

• Rollerblading, rollerskating, and riding a scooter are fun ways to travel outdoors and keep fit at the same time. Don't forget to wear a helmet and some elbow and knee pads for safety.

• Dance! Whether you go out to a club, host a dance party at home or find an online class, dancing gives you a fantastic whole-body workout, tones your muscles, increases stamina, and burns about the same number of calories as jogging. In addition, music causes the release of "happy hormones" that make us feel better.

• Go hiking in the countryside. When you're outdoors enjoying nature and moving your body, you'll be improving your fitness, strength, and mood at the same time. Explore your local area and choose a leisurely saunter or a steep climb—whatever you want.

• Take a friend to the park and throw a frisbee to each other. It will get your heart pumping, increase your speed and agility, and also strengthen your arms and legs. Beware of enthusiastic dogs wanting to join in..!

6 WAYS TO MAKE EXERCISE FUN

Having fun when you exercise will make a huge difference, enabling you to ditch the sofa and reach for your fitness kit on days when you feel tired. Start slowly and build your confidence gradually—don't expect to be super-fit, fast, or flexible straight away.

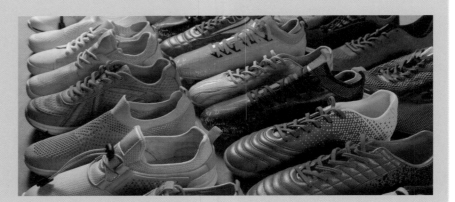

1. Get the right kit

It's amazing how positive you can feel as soon as you put on your fitness gear. As well as choosing colors and styles that you like, your exercise clothes need to be comfortable and lightweight, let you move easily and allow air to circulate and moisture to evaporate. If you're doing higher-intensity exercise, such as running, visit a specialist running store and buy the right pair of running shoes to suit your style. For women doing cardio exercise, a supportive sports bra is essential.

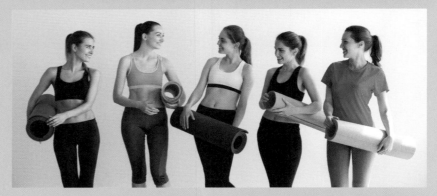

2. Join a class

If you'd like to try something you've never done before—such as yoga or Pilates, for example—take part in a few beginner's classes while you build confidence. Find out what's available in your local area and ask if you might take a look at the facilities on offer. Once you start an exercise class, you may find you are hooked for life!

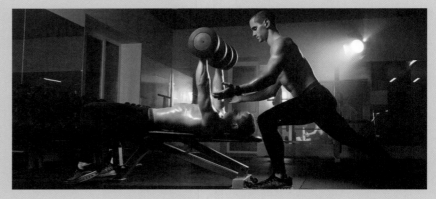

4. Get a tailored program

If you're planning on weight training or doing general exercises in the gym, consider booking a few sessions with a personal trainer. They can devise a program to suit your goals. Be honest if they give you exercises you don't like—giving them feedback will enable them to adapt the program to suit your likes and dislikes.

4. Set yourself an exercise goal

Your goal might be to walk to your local park and back every day, ride your bike on weekends, do yoga three times a week, or run 5 km (3 miles) in eight or ten weeks' time. It might help to make your exercise goal "official" by signing up to do a short run, a sponsored walk, or a mini-triathlon. There's no greater motivation to keep exercising than to know that you've got to get fit by a certain date!

5. Enlist support

Social support is a strong motivator for exercise and can positively influence your success and desire to keep going with it. Tell your family and friends that you are making an effort to be more active and ask them to encourage you to keep up the good work. Better still, start exercising with them! Studies show that couples and families maintain their commitment to keep fit by working out together. This improves health, lowers stress levels, and leads to closer relationships—so it's a win-win situation all round!

6. Make exercise a regular habit

It will take a while for your body to adapt and get fitter, but once exercise becomes a regular part of your routine, it's much easier to maintain. It goes without saying that exercise does not have to take place in a gym. If you're not a gym bunny but prefer walking, running, cycling, or swimming, choose that. And don't let the weather stop you from moving. If it's raining, you can still exercise at home... or take an umbrella and walk around the block!. Find whatever type of exercise you like and keep doing it—it's that simple.

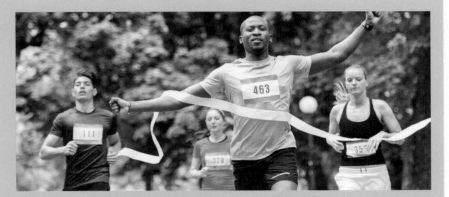

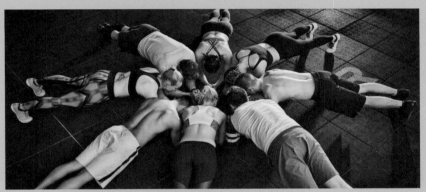

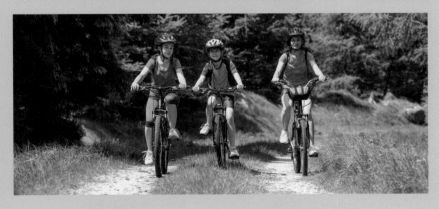

USE YOUR INTUITION

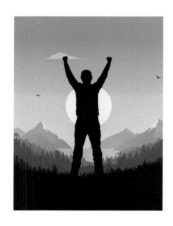

Why stick to a rigid exercise routine when you can reap so many benefits from listening to what your body really needs?

You may have heard of intuitive eating, where you build up your mind-body connection to pick up on feelings of hunger and fullness. Well, intuitive fitness is much the same in that it's the art of tuning in to your body's natural intelligence and listening to physical and emotional cues about what it needs in the moment. The benefits are numerous, including being less likely to injure yourself or get ill from pushing yourself too hard. "Listening in this way gives you the chance to make informed, mindful choices about how your body needs to move," says personal trainer and wellness coach, Holly Goodwin (hollycgoodwin. com). "A number of highly regarded books such as *The Blue Zones* (National Geographic) have looked into the secrets of the world's centenarians and how they've managed to live such a long life. All were active in some way every day, however none of them owned a gym membership or forced themselves to run a certain number of miles each week," says Holly. "Intuitive fitness gives you the opportunity to ask yourself, 'How am I feeling today?'" Once you know how you feel, you can decide which exercise will be best.

STAYING MOTIVATED

"Goals are important and whether you're training for a marathon or just want to be able to do a press-up, it's great to have a target," says Holly. "Many people thrive on structure, and I find most of my clients want routine and accountability and worry that they'll be tempted to ditch exercise altogether if given the choice." However, the flip side of a rigid structure is that you can develop tunnel vision and become disconnected from what your body needs and focus too heavily on what you want to achieve, which isn't the best approach for overall health. "It can also lead to injury if you push your body too hard. As a result, listening to your body is likely to get you closer to your goal in the long run," says Holly. "It's important to note that all movement counts. It's not just the spin class or the gym session—it's your day-to-day commitment to move in a way that feels good and nourishes your body." For those concerned about the temptation to stop exercising altogether and who prefer structure, Holly recommends bringing a more intuitive approach into your current regime. "Do this by continuing to exercise in a way that will help you achieve your goals, but substitute one or two of the days for an intuitive day, where you listen to your body and do what feels best. For example, if you're feeling a little drained and uninspired, instead of running on a treadmill, go for a hike. Or, if you think you might have an injury brewing, take a rest day."

EXERCISE INTUITIVELY
Move in any way that feels nourishing to your body. All types of movement count.

EXERCISING FOR EVERY MOOD

Here are Holly's workout suggestions linked to how you're feeling.

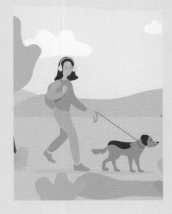

If you're feeling sluggish and lethargic...

Go outdoors! The last thing you need when you feel sluggish is to go to the gym or an indoor class. Load up a podcast and go for a walk—10–15 minutes is all you need. Once you get into the fresh air, the oxygen and your boosted circulation will kick in and you'll feel energized. You might even want to break into a power walk.

If you feel depressed and lacking energy...

Cardio is a must when you feel down, as it helps to boost your endorphins—your "feel-good" hormones. Something I recommend to my clients is jumping on are bounder (a mini trampoline). It can be done at home; bouncing for just 10 minutes can help to detoxify your lymph nodes and boost your energy levels.

If you feel stressed or anxious...

Breathwork is the most important here, and yoga is one of the best workouts for combining both movement and breath. Moving in this relaxed, flowing motion immediately reduces anxiety and strengthens your parasympathetic "rest and digest" nervous system. Moves that require you to stay low and close to the floor can create a feeling of security.

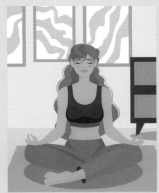

If it's that time of the month or your joints are bothering you...

Whether you're on your period or going through menopause, this is a turbulent and changeable time for your hormones and, as a result, your mood can suffer. Movement is great for relieving symptoms, but it's best to keep it gentle. A cooling swim will get your heart pumping without working up a sweat, or perhaps opt for some stretches. These forms of exercise are great for easing pressure on your joints.

If you feel energized and well rested...

This is a great opportunity to get in some resistance training and high-intensity workouts. High-octane classes are perfect when you're on top of your game. Alternatively, steady cardio workouts, such as running, are also a good option.

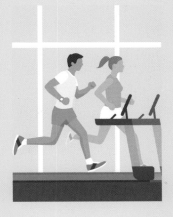

A HEARTY WORKOUT

Cardio is the best choice when it comes to exercising for your heart, and broadening your workout style will offer even more benefits.

Experts agree that when it comes to exercise, cardio (or aerobic) activities are the best sort for your heart. After all, the clue is in the name! But research also suggests that finding a weekly balance between the three main types of exercise—cardio, resistance and flexibility—could bring optimum heart health. "These activities all complement each other," says Chris Allen, senior cardiac nurse with the British Heart Foundation (bhf.org.uk). "So to really reap the health benefits, most people should try to incorporate all three types of exercises into their regime. Try to have a holistic view of your health, and make sure both your diet and your exercise regime are nourishing your body." Here's how...

GET YOUR HEART PUMPING

Cardio activities such as running, brisk walking, rowing, swimming, or cycling are all fabulous for your heart. "Cardiovascular exercise makes the heart stronger and more efficient at pumping blood around the body," says personal trainer Stephen McConville (nuffieldhealth.com). "Regular cardio will lower your resting heart rate and your blood pressure. Having lower blood pressure puts less stress on the circulatory system, meaning you're less likely to develop cardiovascular disease. "Cardiovascular exercise is brilliant, not only

Below: Named after a New York physiologist, the burpee is a full-body exercise in which you go into a squat position with your hands on the ground, kick your feet back into an extended plank position, return your feet into the squat position, then stand up and repeat.

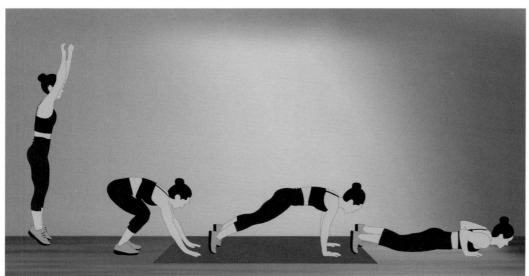

QUICK CARDIO EXERCISES
The following exercises will get your heart going:
• Jumping jacks.
• Running in place, bringing your knees up toward your chest.
• Squat jumps.
• Burpees (squat, jump, and press-up).
• Step-ups.
• Jumping rope.

for the heart itself, but for the systems in which the organ functions. For example, it is known to reduce levels of 'bad cholesterol' LDL, helping you to maintain clean arteries."

BUILD YOUR MUSCLES

Resistance or strength workouts commonly involve weight training, but can include any type of exercise where you lift or pull against some form of resistance. So you might, for example, use the resistance of your own bodyweight to do moves such as press-ups or squats. "Strength exercises will help to keep your blood pressure and blood sugar under control," says Chris. "They're also really useful for managing your weight and building and maintaining good bone health." In fact, static exercises (such as weightlifting) could even improve certain key markers of heart health more than dynamic activities (such as cycling), according to a recent study at the University of Grenada. "Having strong muscles through resistance training will boost your metabolism, helping you burn fat more easily and putting less stress on your heart," says Stephen.

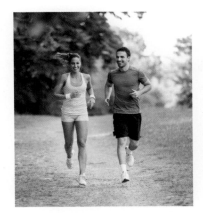
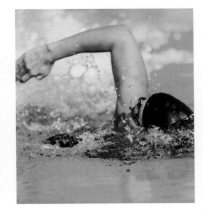

BEND AND STRETCH

Activities that develop flexibility—such as tai chi, yoga and stretching—don't always have much direct impact on your heart, although fast-paced yoga flow classes can get your blood pumping. Nevertheless, by guarding against injury and keeping you supple, flexibility work can help you stay exercising regularly for longer. As such, flexibility is something of an unsung hero when it comes to heart health—plus, by supporting our mental health, it can have further indirect benefits. "Many people who are stressed cope by smoking, drinking alcohol and eating processed foods," says Chris. "You can protect your cardiac fitness by turning to something like yoga instead, as there's a lot of evidence that yoga can help to relieve stress." Risk factors for cardiovascular disease have been shown to improve more in those doing yoga than in those doing no exercise, according to a study published in the *European Journal of Preventative Cardiology*.

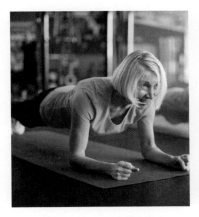
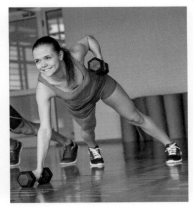
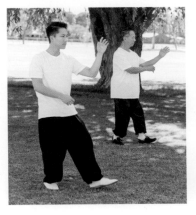
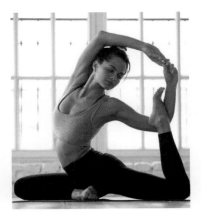

CYCLING

If you're looking for a fantastic and freeing way to give your heart, blood vessels, lungs, and legs a complete workout, cycling has to be high on the list of fun cardio activities to try. Getting on a bike and hitting the open road not only improves your physical fitness, it also has important mental health benefits, from clearing your mind to broadening your social circle. Here's a list of what cycling can do for you:

- Lowers your risk of developing major illnesses, such as heart disease and cancer.
- Improves your lung function.
- Builds muscles in your glutes, hamstrings, quads, and calves, while simultaneously burning fat.
- Helps you to lose weight.
- Strengthens your immune system.
- Saves your joints from high-impact activities (such as running, for example).
- Saves you time when you're traveling and lets you enjoy your surroundings while you get there.
- Helps your navigational and spacial skills.
- Improves your mental wellbeing and helps you to meet like-minded people.

There are plenty of different types of cycling and bikes to try—including road, mountain, track, BMX, cyclo-cross, or even tandem cycling on a bicycle built for two!—so whether you're commuting across town to get to work or going on an epic touring adventure in the mountains, there's sure to be something you'll love.

Note: Don't forget to wear a helmet, take a bottle of water, and check that your bike's bell and safety features are in good working order before you set off.

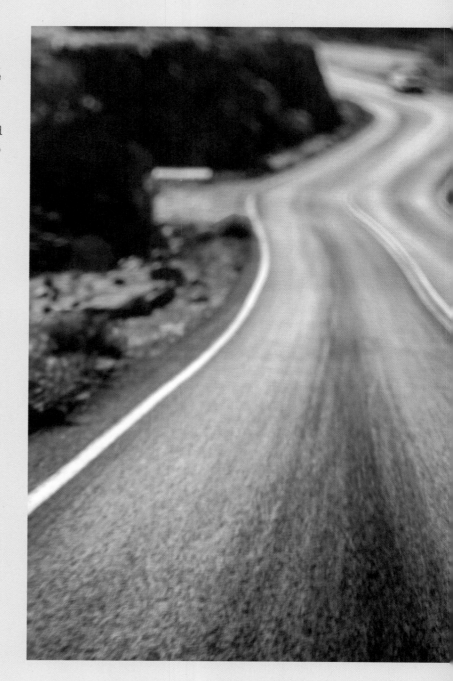

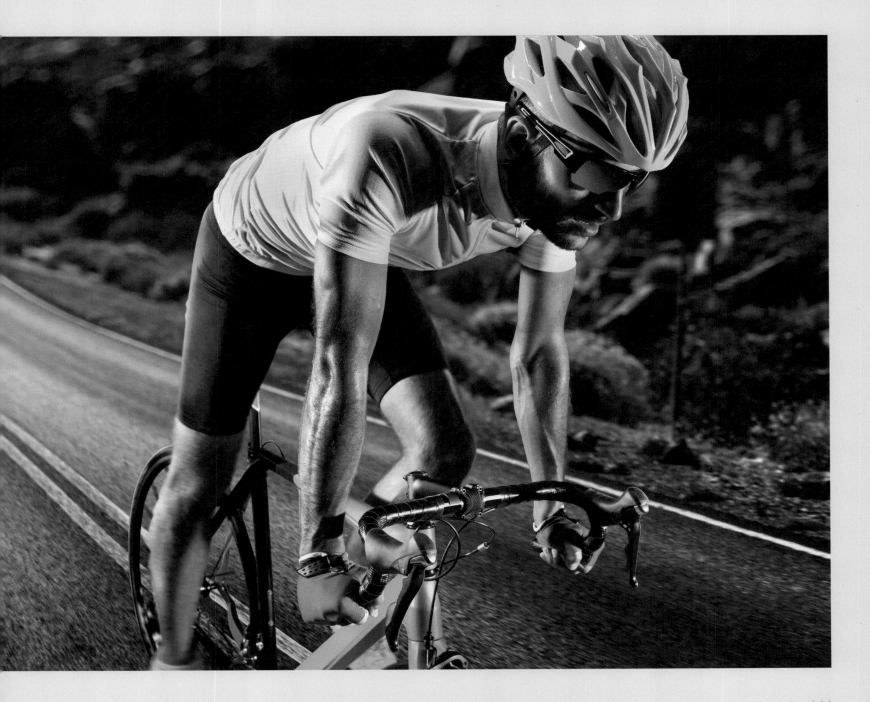

STRETCHING YOUR BOUNDARIES

Whether you're suffering from minor issues or just want to improve your flexibility in general, assisted stretching could be the answer.

As The Beatles once sagely pointed out, we get by with a little help from our friends. But have you ever considered that you might benefit from a (literal) helping hand from someone else? It's easy to neglect stretches or give a cursory nod to tight glutes and calves, but gaining a bit of professional help can work wonders. But what exactly is assisted stretching? In a nutshell, it's when someone else—most likely a personal trainer, physiotherapist, or chiropractor—helps you move more deeply into a stretch.

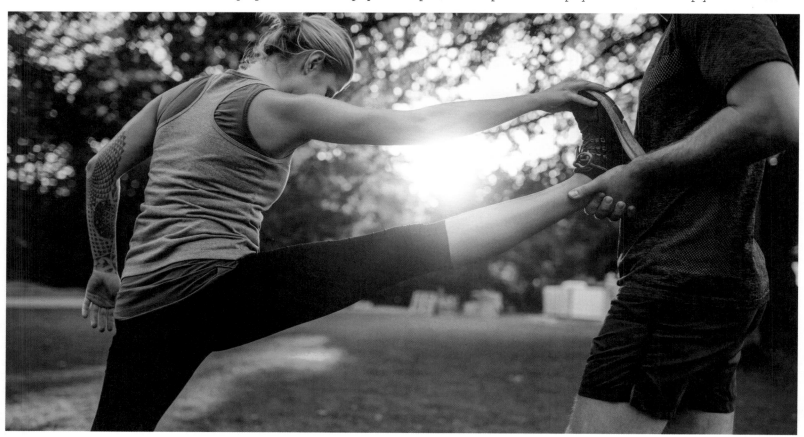

If you've ever seen a physical therapist at the gym leaning over a client who's lying down, helping to press their knee toward their body, you'll get the idea. "The theory is that it helps improve your mobility more quickly than static stretches, and having an expert who knows how to apply pressure safely can take the guesswork out," says Alastair Crew, a personal trainer and Product Head at David Lloyd Gyms. "There are many different techniques and styles, depending on training and preference, but they all work just as well towards the same goal."

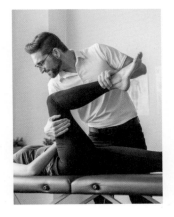

Most stretching will involve you gently contracting and relaxing your muscles while the trainer helps guide your body into slightly deeper movements. It turns out that this gentle encouragement can have a lasting impact. "You're basically tricking your nervous system into increasing your range of motion," says Alastair. "When your body feels unsafe—for example, if it feels that attempting the splits would likely cause injury—it will prevent you from going further. But when it feels safe it will let you move a little more."

There are times when assisted stretching should be used with caution. It probably won't suit people with hypermobility, for example, and if you're injured you should tell your trainer. "There are exercises to help people rehabilitate from injuries or correct postural issues," says Alastair. "If you're injured it might be worth seeking a physical therapist who is a corrective exercise specialist, who can spend a big chunk of the sessions on improving your range of mobility." However, assisted stretching can benefit the majority of people. "It's a nice way to keep up your general body maintenance," says Alastair. And if you're not keen on being touched, it doesn't rule it out as an option—there are alternative methods that trainers can utilise, such as using a foam roller as a barrier between the two of you. The best part? Aside from sometimes feeling intense (but never painful), it's actually quite an enjoyable treatment.

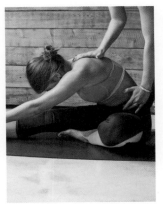

DO-IT-YOURSELF STRETCHING
While it's not advisable to try assisted stretching with a friend rather than a professional, there are some self-massages and stretching techniques that can achieve similar results.

Foam rolling: "This is about myofascial release," says Alistair. "Roll along your muscles until you find a tender spot, stop, and hold the pressure for 20–30 seconds, when you should feel a release. On a scale of 1 to 10, with 1 being feeling nothing and 10 bringing tears to your eyes, you're looking for about a 7. This can help you see a 50–70 percent reduction in sensitivity, which should help you move more easily."

Power plate: If your gym has a Power plate (or other version of this body vibration tool), you can use it for increased mobility. "Stand on it and do your usual static stretches—the vibrations and slight instability will help you travel deeper into the position and reduce discomfort, while holding the handles will help you into the stretches safely," says Alastair.

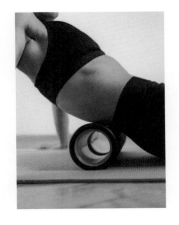

WORK OUT INDOORS

In many ways, the COVID pandemic and its many restrictions have raised our awareness of the importance of staying active. If you can't get to the gym or your favorite local exercise class, there are plenty of ways to create a mini gym at home with just a few bits of equipment.

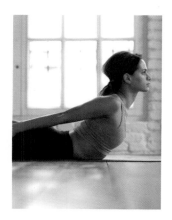

EXERCISE MAT

An exercise mat helps you do floorwork, yoga, Pilates, and stretching. The benefit of a good mat is that it's very soft and spongy. This helps to cushion your back, especially when you have to lie on a hard floor.

For good posture, try the **Lying Prone Cobra**: Lie face down on the mat with your hands by your sides. Keeping your head in alignment with your neck, lift your chest off the ground slightly by squeezing your shoulder blades together and down. Hold for 2 seconds, then lower. Repeat 10 times.

DUMBBELLS

These are extremely versatile—you can do thousands of exercises with them! Dumbbells also highlight any imbalances in your body, such as your right arm being weaker than your left, which you don't get to find out by using fixed equipment in the gym.

For toned shoulders, try the **Curl and Press**: With dumbbells by your sides, bend your elbows to bring the weights up to your shoulders, then push them above your head. Slowly lower the dumbbells back to the start, in toward your shoulders first, then curling down. Repeat 10 times.

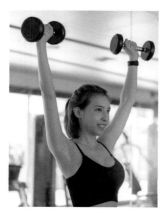

EXERCISE BALL

A Swiss ball is cheap and can be used for multiple exercises. Whether you add resistance such as dumbbells or just use your bodyweight, it can be challenging for your body in various ways.

For a toned abdomen, try the **Jackknife**: Go into a press-up position with your shins on the ball. Keeping your back straight, pull your knees toward your chest. Stop if you feel it in your back—this should work your legs and stomach. Repeat 10 times.

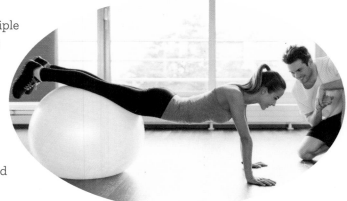

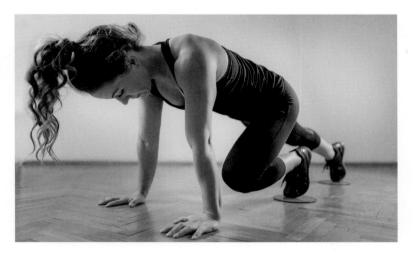

GLIDING DISCS

These are a novel way of exercising without lots of equipment. They work your core muscles as they create instability, so you have to work hard while your limbs are sliding.

To really work your stomach muscles and strenghten your core, try **Mountain Climbers**: In a press-up position, and on a surface that will slip, put your feet on each disc with one forward and one back. Swap leg positions forward and backward for 1 minute.

ADJUSTABLE WEIGHT BENCH

An adjustable step is great if you want a bench on a budget. You can use it for a variety of step-up moves, but it's also very useful for resistance training.

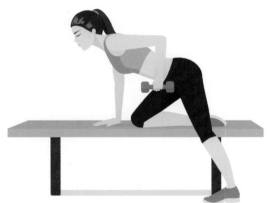

For sculpted arms, try the **Single Arm Row**: Kneel on one end of the step with your right knee, and place your right hand onto the other end of the step. Keep your left foot on the floor. With your left hand, lift a weight upward, keeping your back straight and your elbow tucked into your body. Pause, then slowly lower the weight to the floor. Repeat 10 times.

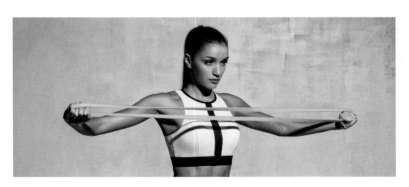

RESISTANCE BANDS

Often used in the field of rehabilitation, resistance bands can help you not only work your muscles but also stretch. There are different thicknesses depending on the activity and outcome you want.

Slumping in front of the TV leads to stooped posture. Counteract this with the **Chest Stretch**: Hold a resistance band at either end out in front of you. Keeping your arms straight, take each arm out to the side and back behind you as far as you can. Repeat 10 times.

15-MINUTE WORKOUT

Many of us give up on our fitness goals when life gets busy, and we think we just don't have the time to work out. Short workouts, however, can be highly effective, as long as you work hard and do them regularly.

Try this 15-minute workout you can do from home. You only need two medium/heavy dumbbells. Perform each exercise as a circuit for 35 seconds, have 25 seconds' rest, and then repeat the same exercise for another set (with the same intervals) before moving onto the next exercise.

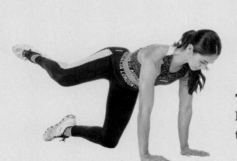

FIRE HYDRANT (*left*)
Good for your glutes

- Start on all fours, hands directly under your shoulders, hips directly over your knees.
- Lift your right knee out to the side, squeezing your right glute to lift the leg to 90 degrees, or as far as your mobility allows.
- Lower and repeat, then do the other leg.

TIPS: To make it harder, pulse four times at the top of the leg lift. Make sure you keep your back flat and don't rotate your hips throughout the sets. Use a slow and controlled movement.

WEIGHTED GLUTE BRIDGES (*right*)
Good for your glutes and hamstrings

- Lie on your back, placing one dumbbell across your hips. Place you heels near to your bottom.
- Lift your hips, squeezing the glutes at the top. Create a straight line from your knees to your chest.
- Advanced version: Change the tempo—either do fast repetitions or slow the pace to focus on squeezing and holding the glutes at the top of each rep.

TIP: Don't over-arch your spine.

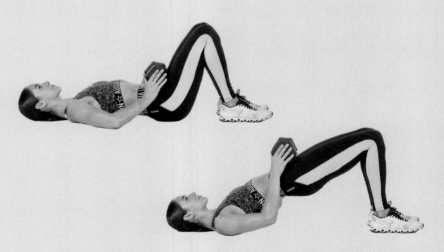

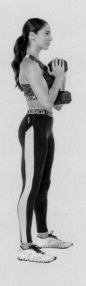
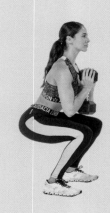

GOBLET SQUAT (*left*)

Good for building strength, stability, mobility, and flexibility, works your lower body (glutes, quads, hamstrings, calves, and abdominals) and increases flexibility of your ankles and feet

- Holding one dumbbell to your chest with both hands, stand with your feet shoulder-width apart, toes pointing slightly out. Bend at the hips and knees, keeping your back straight, looking forward.
- Keep your weight over your heels, sit in the squat for a second, then push through your heels back up to standing.
- Advanced version: Add 4 pulses at the bottom of the squat or tempo squat, 3 counts down, 1 drive up.

TIPS: Do not hunch your shoulders. Ensure your back is straight throughout.

TRICEPS PUSH-UPS (*right*)

Good for your chest, triceps, shoulders, and core

- Start in high plank, shoulders directly over your hands. Lower your body to the floor, keeping your elbows pinned to your sides.
- Ensure your core is braced, squeezing your belly button toward your spine throughout.
- Advanced version: Add 4 pulses at the bottom of the press-up.

TIP: Don't let your hips sink to the floor through the press-up; ensure a flat back through each repetition.

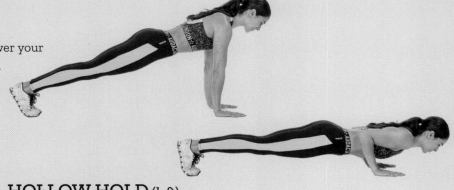

HOLLOW HOLD (*left*)

Good for your abdominals and obliques

- Lie on your back with your arms reaching above your head, your biceps tight to your ears.
- Place your legs straight out in front of you. Lift your head, upper back, and legs a few inches off the floor, pushing your lower back into the floor.
- Imagine yourself as a banana shape, keeping your core, legs, and arms tight throughout.

TIPS: Squeeze your belly button down toward your spine throughout, to ensure there is no gap between your back and the floor. Modify by raising your legs higher and/or bending slightly at your knees.

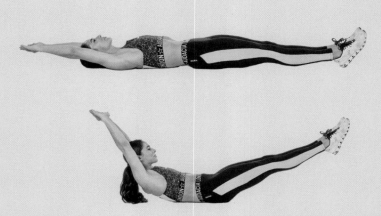

HAMSTRING WALKOUTS (below)

Good for your hamstrings and glutes

- Lie on your back, placing your heels close to your bottom.
- Lift your hips, squeezing the glutes at the top. Lift your toes off the floor so you are resting on your heels. Create a straight line from your knees to your chest.
- Walk your heels away from your body until your legs are straight, ensuring your hips are lifted throughout.
- Walk your feet back to the start position. Repeat.

TIP: Do small walkout movements and ensure your glutes are squeezed, with your hips lifted throughout.

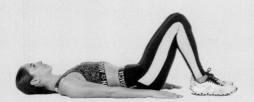 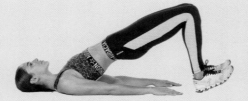 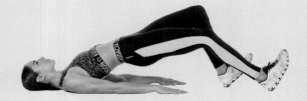

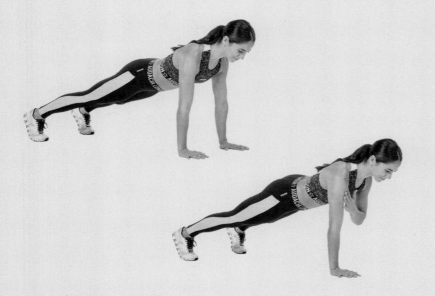

PLANK SHOULDER TAPS (left)

Good for your shoulders and core

- Start in a high plank position, your hands directly under your shoulders, and your feet hip-distance apart.
- Keeping your head, back, and hips in a straight line, tap one hand to the opposite shoulder.

TIPS: Ensure your core and glutes are engaged throughout each rep. Do not let your hips dip to the floor. Keep your back flat enough to rest a drink on it!

HOW TO INCORPORATE MOVEMENT INTO YOUR DAY

Even during a hectic week when you don't have time for the gym, you can still fit in short amounts of exercise throughout your day—and these short amounts all combine together to make a big difference in the long run.

- When traveling to work, get off your train or bus a bit earlier than usual or park your car a little further away, and walk the rest of the way. Not only will you get more exercise, you'll also benefit from the fresh air and sunshine.

- If you sit at a desk, set a timer to go off every 30 minutes, to remind you to stand up, do some stretching exercises, or go for a little walk.

- Take phone calls standing up or while walking around the room.

- Go for a walk at lunchtime—explore your surroundings, visit an art gallery, jog around a nearby park, browse in some shops, or just see how far you can walk in the time available.

- If your building has an elevator, take the stairs instead.

- Try an adjustable standing desk and switch from standing to sitting—and vice versa—throughout your working day.

- Home activities such as housework, gardening, and walking the dog are all good exercise, too.

ARMED FOR SUCCESS

Here are three good exercises for giving you shaped, toned, and sculpted arms. You can do them almost anywhere!

Perform three to four sets, aiming for 10–12 repetitions of each exercise. The only kit needed is a resistance band and a chair or bench. The last few reps of each set should feel challenging. If not, increase the weight. Use a slow and controlled movement when doing the exercise, and make sure you feel your arms working. Avoid swinging your back on the biceps exercises. Keep your upper body still.

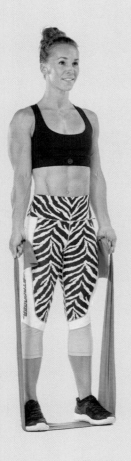
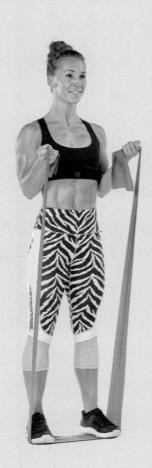

BICEPS CURL (left)

With a resistance band

- Holding onto each end of the resistance band, step your feet onto the middle of the band to secure it to the floor.
- To begin, have your arms extended down by your sides, palms facing forward.
- With your elbows pinned to your sides, bring your hands upward toward your chest, stopping a few inches before your chest or elbows start to leave your sides.

TIP: Don't swing your hips into the movement; ensure your core is braced the entire time. The movement should be generated from driving your hands forward and upward.

TRICEPS KICKBACK *(right)*

With a resistance band

- Place the resistance band in one hand, then step onto the middle of the band to secure it to the floor. Once secured, hinge at your hips and lower your chest 45 degrees toward the floor, keeping your back flat with your other heel off the ground (split-stance style).
- Rest your non-handle hand on your hip.
- Using your other arm, bring your elbow up and pin it to your side to make a 90-degree angle from your shoulder to your elbow to your hand.
- Extend your hand back behind you. Adjust the length of the band as needed, to feel the resistance in the back of your arm.
- Repeat 12 reps and perform two sets on each arm.

TIP: Don't let your lower back arch in either movement. Ensure your core is braced and your hips are tucked under. The movement is generated from driving your hands.

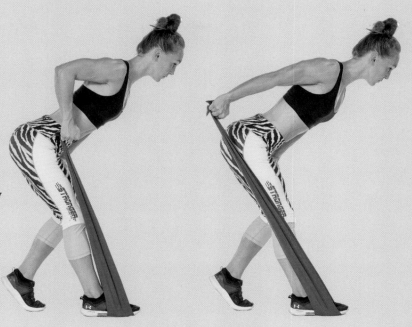

TRICEPS DIP *(left)*

With a chair or bench

- Position your hands shoulder-width apart with your arms straight, facing away from your chair or bench with your legs in front of you (straight or at 90 degrees).
- Brace your core and lower your body by bending your elbows backward, keeping them tight to your body.
- Pause at the bottom, then press back up, maintaining a tight core.
- Advanced option: With straight legs resting on your heels, lift one foot off the floor.

TIP: Don't lock out your arms at the top.

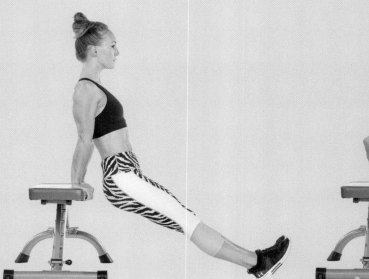

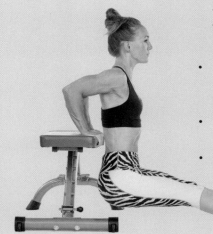

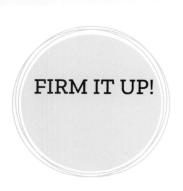

FIRM IT UP!

It's important to tone your buttocks muscles, as lazy glutes can lead to poor posture and even hip injuries. A peachy rear is an added bonus!

Your glutes are one of the most important and powerful muscles in your body. Located around your pelvis, they are responsible for many actions, including kicking, pulling your legs back when you run, or going from sitting to standing. You use them every day so in theory they should be strong, and yet many people end up with lazy glute muscles because they lead a sedentary lifestyle. If you tend to sit a lot, either at a desk, in a car, or on the sofa at home, this leads to tight hips and lower back. Your glutes, on the other hand, start lengthening, weakening and, essentially, going to sleep because they're stretched and underused. This means that when you do perform a move, whether it's squats or lunges in the gym or simply picking up a heavy box or tying your shoes, instead of your glutes doing most of the work, your hip flexors and lower back take over as they've become accustomed to doing so. Think of braces for teeth: they slowly and gradually move your teeth over a period of time by pushing them into a new position. Muscles are obviously softer than teeth, and if they are held in set positions over a long period, they too change in position as well as size and length.

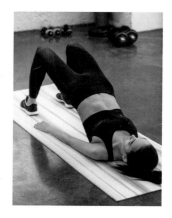

BETTER FOR FITNESS

So how do sleepy glutes affect sporting and exercise performance? If you're into cycling, for instance, you'll be mainly working your quadriceps—the large muscles in your thighs. And, because you're in a seated position, you'll never fully engage your glutes as your legs never extend all the way behind you. So, make sure you focus on lengthening your quads between cycling sessions by doing stretches, and also strengthening your glutes. Rowing, canoeing, and anything where you are sitting down will also cause the same problem. If you do happen to spend the day commuting and then sitting in an office, it's best to avoid using the rower and bike when in the gym. Instead, aim to elongate your body rather than compounding the problem of being hunched over. Being in a more upright position gives your glutes a better chance of working properly. So, for your cardio warm-up, stick to the step machine and treadmill. Then move on to the exercises outlined over the page—you'll be in the running for rear of the year in no time!

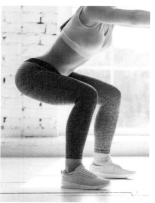

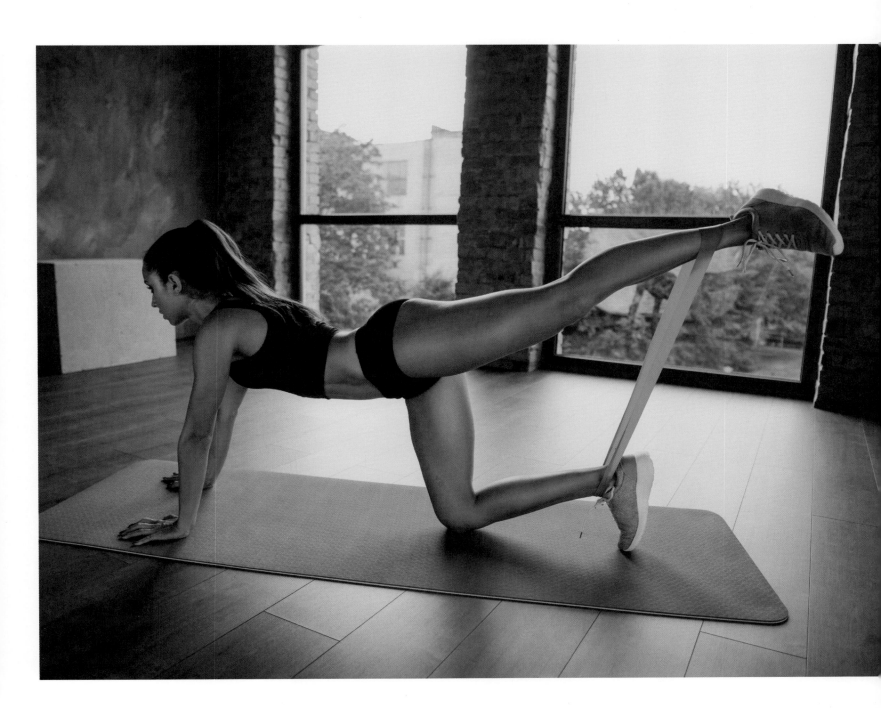

THE POWER OF THREE

Everyone has heard of the gluteus maximus—the largest muscle in your buttocks—but the medius and minimus are just as important. Your gluteus medius runs from your hip joint down to the top of your thigh bone. This is the muscle that's in action when you're doing side leg raises. The gluteus minimus is the smallest of the three, and also runs from the side of your hipbone to your femur but underneath the glute medius. It is used when you do a hip extension, for example, kicking your leg back behind you. These three aren't the only muscles in your bottom and hip area—there are lots of smaller stabilizing ones—but they are the key to doing any kind of glute-shaping workout.

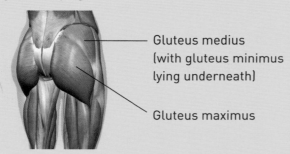

Gluteus medius (with gluteus minimus lying underneath)

Gluteus maximus

How to assess your glute muscles

This quick test—called a modified Thomas test—helps you work out whether your glute muscles are working well.

1. Lie on your bed with your legs hanging off the edge (if your feet easily touch the floor, find something higher to lie on, as you want your legs to dangle freely).
2. Pull one knee in tightly toward your chest and hold it there with both hands.
3. Notice the position of your outstretched leg: the knee should ideally be lower than the hip. If, instead, your knee is higher than your hip, it indicates tightness in your hip flexors, which can mean weak glutes.

4 EXERCISES FOR GLUTES

These exercises are effective at working all three main buttocks muscles: the glutes maximus, medius, and minimus. It's best to do them in this order as it allows full activation of your muscles. Build up stability in this way before moving on to harder exercises or doing them with weights.

1. BRIDGE LIFT

- Lie on your back with your feet flat on the floor close to your bottom. Your arms should both be straight down on the ground beside you.
- Activate your glutes to push your hips up toward the ceiling, being careful not to go so far that your chest pushes into your jaw. Aim to keep your shoulders and upper back still on the ground so it's really only your lower body that's up (this will also make it harder work for your glutes).
- Squeeze and hold at the top for a few seconds, then lower back down.
- Do 20 repetitions.

Progression

Once you can comfortably do this, you can make the exercise harder by picking one foot up off the floor when your hips are in the raised position. Make sure you keep your hips level when you do this—they'll want to dip down on the side you lift, but aim to keep them flat.

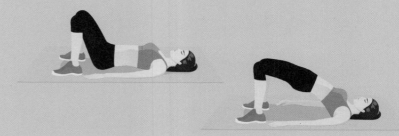

2. CLAMSHELL

- Lie on your side with your legs stacked one on top of the other.
- Put your top arm down on the floor in front of you for support. Keeping your feet together, lift your top knee up as much as you can, squeeze your glute at the top, then lower back down.
- Do 20 repetitions, then repeat on other leg

Progression
Try this with your top leg straight throughout the movement.

3. SINGLE-LEG REACH

- Stand on one leg, then, keeping your back flat, tip your body forward towards the floor, raising your other leg out behind you—a bit like a seesaw.
- Touch the knee of your supporting leg, then, squeezing the glutes on that leg, push back up to standing.
- Perform this 20 times, then do the same on the other leg.

Progression
Hold a weight in the hand that's reaching downward.

4. DEEP SQUAT

- Stand with your feet shoulder-width apart.
- Raise your arms in front of you, parallel to the floor. Keeping your chest up, bend your legs from the hips and sit as low as you can with your back flat—ideally your bottom will touch your heels. If you can't get that low, put a thick book under each heel to raise them slightly.
- Squeeze your buttocks and push back up to the start position.
- Repeat 20 times.

Progression
Pause at the bottom for three seconds on each repetition.

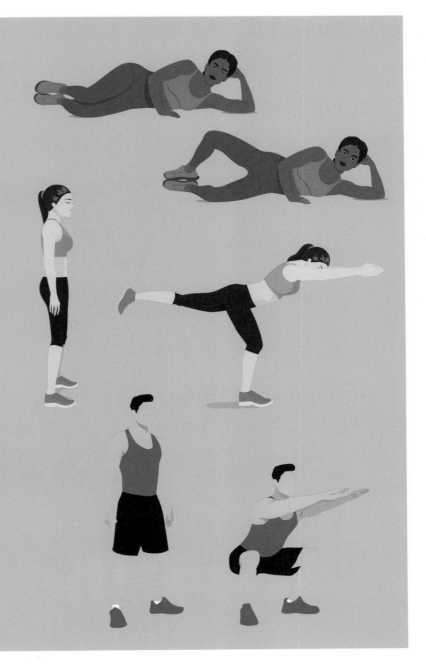

WHAT'S YOUR YOGA TYPE?

Yoga develops strength, balance, and flexibility, but without the "no pain, no gain" mentality. It's all about the union between the body, mind, and spirit, aiming to create feelings of lightness, ease, and relaxation. There are many different types of yoga, from passive stretching to fast-paced sequences, so there's a yoga class for everyone.

HATHA

Hatha refers to the physical practice of yoga: postures (asanas) as opposed to the other branches of yoga, which include bhakti (devotion) and karma (selfless service). So, all the following are forms of hatha yoga. When you see hatha yoga on a class timetable, it usually means a gentle class that includes the traditional asanas common to many types of yoga, as well as pranayama (breathing exercises).

ASHTANGA

Sometimes called power yoga, ashtanga is energetic and fast-paced, with a progressive sequence of asanas synchronized with the breath. Each pose is held for only five breaths and energy is channelled through the body using bandhas (locks). The series produces intense internal heat, designed to tone and purify the body.

BEFORE YOU BEGIN
At the beginning of each yoga class, a good teacher will ask you if you have any injuries or conditions they need to know about, and will offer you modifications to the poses.

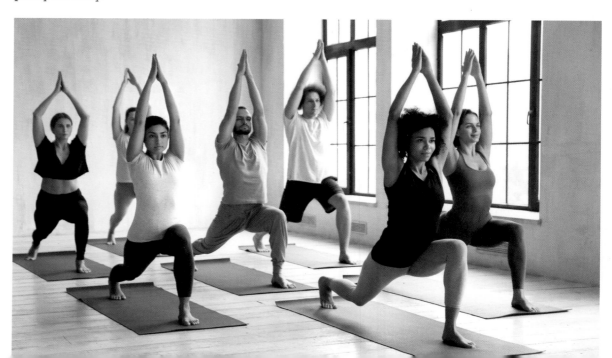

VINYASA

Vinyasa means "breath linked to movement," where every movement is linked with an in-breath and out-breath. Classes called "vinyasa flow" are influenced by ashtanga and move from one pose to the next without pausing.

BIKRAM

Developed by Bikram Choudhury in the 1970s, Bikram classes are sweaty and demanding. The 90-minute sessions follow a format of 26 postures, performed twice, and two breathing exercises, held in rooms heated to 40° C (105° F) with 40 percent humidity. Working in the heat elevates your heart rate, warms your muscles, and is said to help your body relax, improve your breathing, and focus your mind, allowing you to deepen further into the poses and increase your flexibility. Speak to your doctor before doing a class, as exercising in the heat raises the heart rate and is not suitable for people with certain heart conditions, high or low blood pressure, or those taking some medications. Don't do Bikram yoga when pregnant.

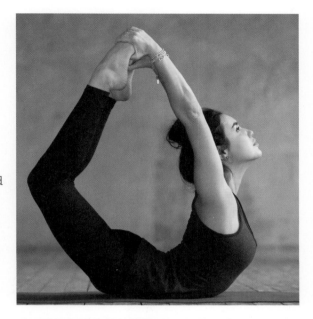

RESTORATIVE

First developed by B.K.S. Iyengar, restorative yoga restores the balance of body and mind so the body can heal itself. The focus is on deep relaxation, breathwork, mindfulness, and opening the body through passive stretching using props and adapted asanas, such as gentle backbends, light twists, and seated forward folds. Blocks, straps, blankets, and bolsters are used to support your body and aid comfort so you can hold asanas for longer and let go fully—you may only do five or six poses in a 60-minute class.

IYENGAR

Named after its founder, Iyengar yoga focuses on precise postural alignment of the body in asanas and breath control, and follows specific, progressive sequences which include more than 200 classical poses and 14 pranayama. The idea is that if the breath and body are aligned, then the mind, emotions, and senses become balanced, too. Using props, poses are held for longer than in many other types of yoga, with the teacher helping to correct misalignments while you're in the pose.

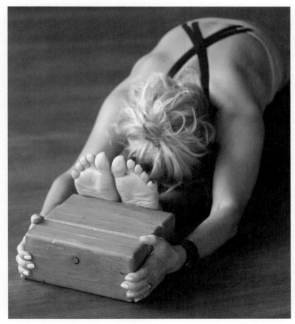

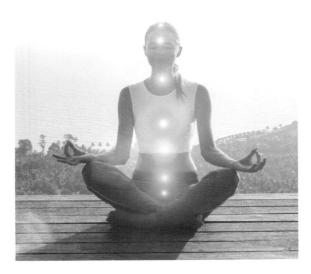

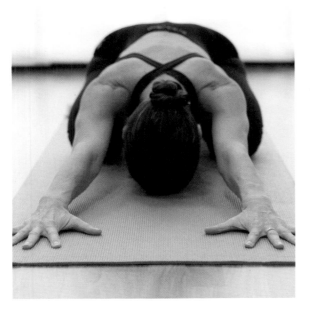

KUNDALINI

Through postures, sound, and breath, kundalini yoga aims to build spiritual awareness by freeing the kundalini, or serpent energy, coiled in the base of the spine and drawing it up the body through the seven chakras. Vigorous asanas, dynamic breathing, chanting, and meditation combine in a kundalini class. With its roots in the tantric yoga tradition, kundalini was brought to the West by Yogi Bhajan in the late 1960s.

SIVANANDA

Named after Swami Sivananda who founded a yoga ashram in Rishikesh in the 1930s, this meditative method focuses on achieving optimal health and spiritual growth through five principles: asana (concentrating on 12 carefully chosen postures, called the Rishikesh series), pranayama, relaxation, vegetarianism, meditation, and positive thinking.

JIVAMUKTI

Probably the hippest form of yoga you'll find, Jivamukti encompasses physical, ethical, and spiritual practice, with classes including vigorous vinyasa-style asanas, music, chanting, and meditation. Founded by Sharon Gannon and David Life in 1984, jivamukti is informed by the ancient Yoga Sutras written by Sage Patanjali and emphasizes compassion toward all beings. Its five tenets are ahimsa (kindness and non-violence), bhakti (devotion), dhyana (meditation), nada (deep listening), and shastra (scripture), with enlightenment or "oneness of being" as the ultimate goal.

YIN

Designed to help you sit longer and feel more comfortable in meditation, slow and gentle yin yoga classes involve variations of seated and supine poses, held for three to five minutes. This slow and passive method allows deeper stretching of the connective tissue and fascia around the muscles and joints. In has its roots in the Taoist tradition, and the opposing forces of yin and yang. Yang movement is vigorous and energetic, working large muscle groups and generating heat in your body, while yin relaxes the muscles and cools the body. English names are often used for the poses instead of Sanskrit, such as butterfly, sleeping swan, or twisted roots.

10 YOGA POSES

There are many different yoga poses, and they can be categorized into five types: standing, balancing, backbends, seated, and resting. Don't be overwhelmed by them or think you'll never be able to do them—if you woke up this morning and stretched your arms above your head, you've already done a yoga pose today! The different poses are designed to help a particular part of your body, such as your abdominals, arms, hamstrings, hips, knees, lower back, or thighs. This table shows ten well-known poses to get you started.

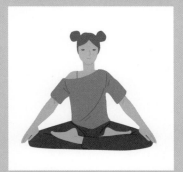

1. Lotus

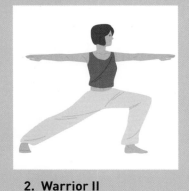

2. Warrior II

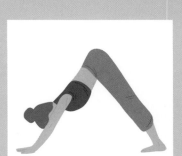

3. Downward Dog

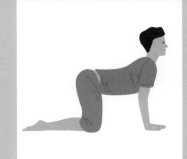

4. Cow

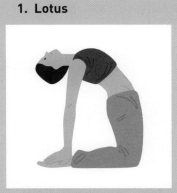

5. Camel

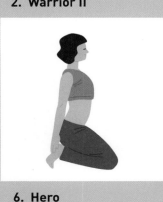

6. Hero

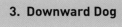

7. Plow

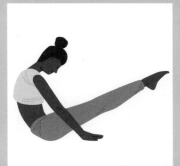

8. Boat

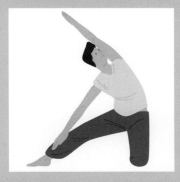

9. Gate

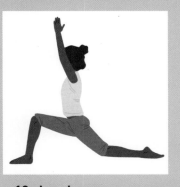

10. Low Lunge

PILATES

If you enjoy yoga, you might also want to look at Pilates, another low-impact exercise. While yoga involves holding static positions, with Pilates you adopt a position and then challenge your core by moving your arms or legs. This is thought to aid recovery after injury, as well as improving posture and strength.

Pilates got its name from its inventor, the early 20th-century German physical trainer Joseph Pilates. He described his exercises as "contrology"—the art of controlled movements—and developed them from looking at animals such as cats. According to Joseph, "Normal muscles should function in much the same manner as do the muscles of animals. How they are constantly stretching and relaxing, twisting, squirming, turning, climbing, wrestling, and fighting." His system emphasized the need for this constant stretching and relaxing.

Joseph also described eight major functional movements that decline with age: walking/gait, sit-to-stand, reaching, bending down, calf strength, dynamic balance (balancing through space while moving), posture (also while in movement and in various spinal shapes), and contralateral movement (exercising muscles on opposite sides of the body simultaneously). Pilates helps with all of these, and some exercises even work to improve all eight at the same time!

> "Generally speaking, yoga is much more about flexibility and stability; Pilates is strength and stability." Prof. Greg Whyte, former Olympian and leading authority on sports science

DID YOU KNOW?
Pilates is suitable for everyone, regardless of age, gender, size, or fitness level, and the only equipment you need is a mat for support. Many professional athletes and dancers include Pilates as part of their fitness routines.

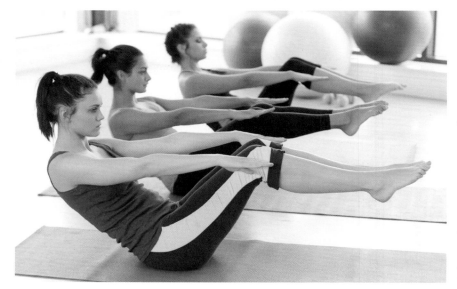

Left: Pilates works your core, also known as your "powerhouse"—the middle of your body, from the base of your rib cage to the base of your buttocks. This includes the muscles of your lower back, abdominals, hips, glutes, inner thighs, and pelvic floor. To function most effectively, your powerhouse works in sync with your breath.

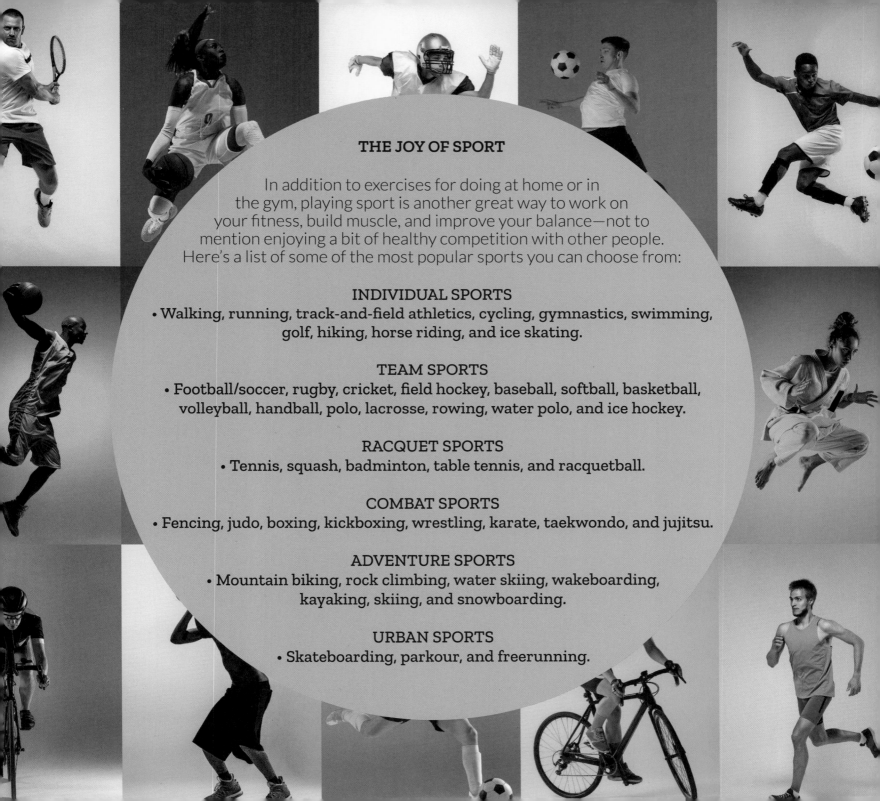

THE JOY OF SPORT

In addition to exercises for doing at home or in the gym, playing sport is another great way to work on your fitness, build muscle, and improve your balance—not to mention enjoying a bit of healthy competition with other people. Here's a list of some of the most popular sports you can choose from:

INDIVIDUAL SPORTS
• Walking, running, track-and-field athletics, cycling, gymnastics, swimming, golf, hiking, horse riding, and ice skating.

TEAM SPORTS
• Football/soccer, rugby, cricket, field hockey, baseball, softball, basketball, volleyball, handball, polo, lacrosse, rowing, water polo, and ice hockey.

RACQUET SPORTS
• Tennis, squash, badminton, table tennis, and racquetball.

COMBAT SPORTS
• Fencing, judo, boxing, kickboxing, wrestling, karate, taekwondo, and jujitsu.

ADVENTURE SPORTS
• Mountain biking, rock climbing, water skiing, wakeboarding, kayaking, skiing, and snowboarding.

URBAN SPORTS
• Skateboarding, parkour, and freerunning.

YOUR 7-DAY PLAN

Want to put all the pieces together? Follow this plan and you'll be getting a good mix of exercise all week long.

MONDAY

BODYWEIGHT RESISTANCE

Kick the week off with a bodyweight resistance workout. Start with squats, press-ups, forward lunges, sideways lunges, and double leg raises (lying on your back). This routine should work all the major muscles in your legs, hips, back, abdomen, chest, shoulders, and arms. Do each exercise 10 or 15 times and repeat each set three times. To get the most health benefits, you need to finish each set feeling you'd struggle to complete another repetition—you should be a little sweaty and out of breath! It's up to you how long you rest between each set, but you can take up to a minute.

TUESDAY

FLEXIBILITY

Time to combine some strength and flexibility exercises at a relaxing but super-conditioning yoga or Pilates class. You could also add power walking to your class, to rack up some more activity minutes for the week.

WEDNESDAY

CARDIO

The middle of the week—"hump day"—is a great time to pack in some cardiovascular exercise, and there's nothing easier or more inspiring than lacing up your trainers for a run. If you can bring a friend along, that's even better, but make sure you're running at a pace where you can't say more than a few words without pausing for breath. Try to incorporate some hill and interval training by challenging yourself to sprint between lampposts and trees. If you struggle to run for a full half hour, then don't worry, you can power walk whenever you need to.

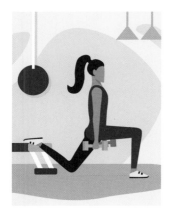

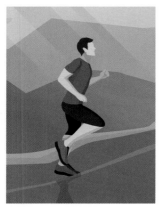

THURSDAY

REST

It's a rest day—and you've earned it. Your heart, mind, and joints will thank you for staying mobile, though, so try to add some walking and stretching into your day.

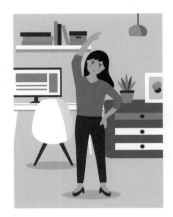

FRIDAY

STRENGTH TRAINING

Hit the gym (or your living room) for a strength workout, using medium dumbbells. Try a round of press-ups, bent over rows, chest presses, and squats (with dumbbells on your shoulders, if you can). Do three sets of 10–15 repetitions each, with no more than 60 seconds of rest in between. If you are at all unsure how to do any of these moves, check with a personal trainer, or join a strength class at your local gym. You could also repeat Monday's workout, which will give you heart-conditioning resistance boost.

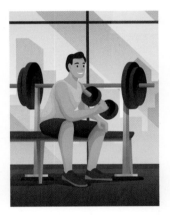

SATURDAY

CARDIO

It's the weekend, so celebrate with some joyful cardio! The key thing here is to make sure you go for something that you truly enjoy. Swimming is an incredible whole-body workout, which torches calories and develops your cardio-respiratory fitness without putting pressure on your joints. Because you have to cut through the resistance of the water, it will also tone and strengthen your body at the same time. It's tempting to stick to a leisurely breaststroke, but make sure you do backstroke and front crawl, too. See if you can introduce a few swim sprints, perhaps once every 10 lengths.

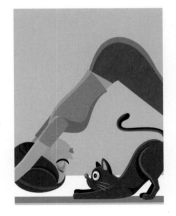

SUNDAY

FLEXIBILITY

While Sunday is traditionally a rest day, incorporating some yoga or Pilates, with a focus on relaxation, is a great way to end your week.

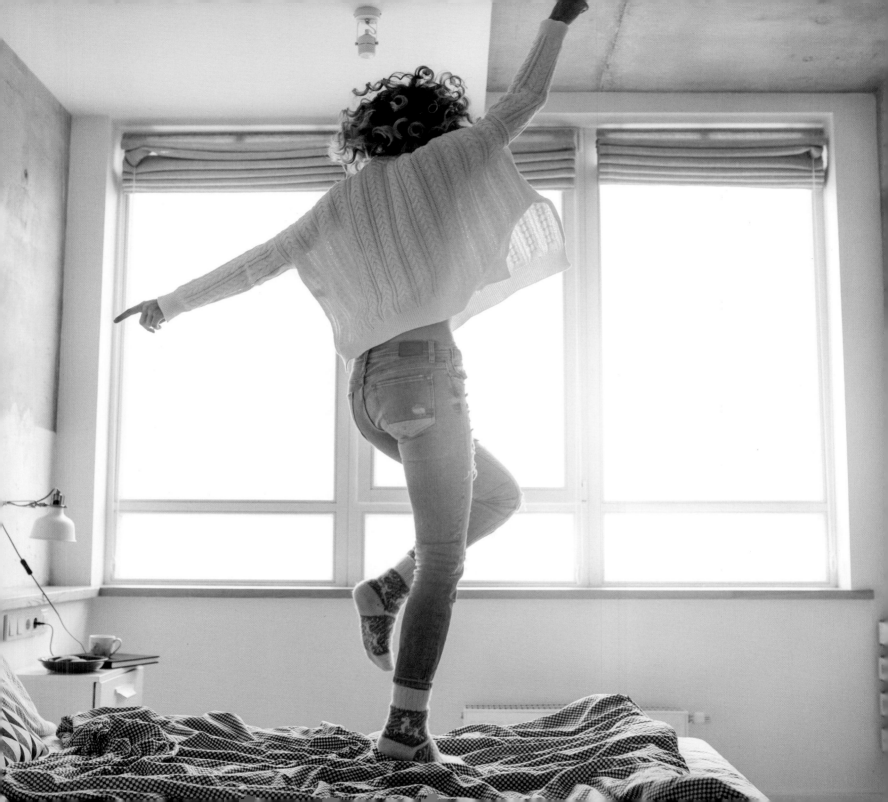

5
HEALTH MATTERS

Take charge of your physical wellbeing with our do-it-yourself tips and expert advice to address common health worries. We start by looking at our spiritual needs and then show how to halt migraines, reduce back pain, steer clear of COVID-19 and other viruses, and combat type 2 diabetes. There is information about men and women's health issues, becoming a parent, and how to get a good night's sleep, and the chapter ends with some complementary and alternative therapies that will help you feel energized and revitalized.

SPIRITUAL SELF-CARE

When looking after our health and wellbeing, it's important for us to connect to our true inner selves. Spiritual self-care has a unique meaning for each of us, but there are universal benefits for all.

Spiritual self-care essentially means doing activities that nurture your spirit and allow you to think bigger than yourself. For some, this may involve religion—for example, attending a place of worship, going to religious services, studying religious text, or simply quiet prayer at home. For others, it may involve a combination of many of the ideas we've discussed in previous chapters, such as meditation, breathwork, yoga, or going for a walk in nature. Whatever activities you choose (see opposite for some ideas), the point is to dedicate time for self-reflection. Studies have shown that working on our spiritual life has many health benefits. Here are a few:

- Gives us a sense of purpose or belonging.
- Improves our relationships and connections with other people.
- Diminishes our feelings of isolation and loneliness.
- Helps us to find out what makes us happy.
- Enhances our feelings of oneness and universality.
- Deepens our relationship with our inner self and increases our connection with our own intuition.
- Helps us to experience more inner peace, tranquility, and a feeling of groundedness.

> "Spiritual self-care is any ritual of practice to further your connection to your higher self, the real you, who you are as an individual without any ego or pretense."
> Carley Schweet, self-care author

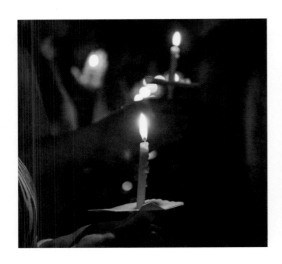
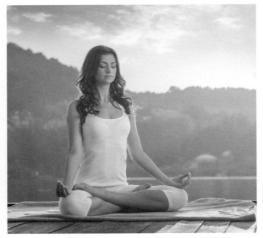
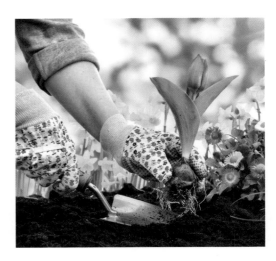

IDEAS FOR CARING FOR
YOUR SPIRIT

Here are a few ways you might look after your spiritual needs. You'll probably be able to think of many more, according to your interests—the right ones will feel intuitive and natural to you.

• Attend a place of worship, talk with a spiritual advisor, read a spiritual or religious book, participate in a healing circle, pray, practice gratitude, or write down a daily list of affirmations.

• Meditate and do some deep breathing exercises, yoga, or Pilates.

• Try sound healing therapy, in which you are immersed in the sound of Tibetan singing bowls, gongs, tuning forks, and drums. The vibrations synchronize your brain waves, relaxing your mind, body, and spirit.

• Go for a walk in nature and notice the sights, smells and sounds around you—the sky, clouds, trees, flowers, birds, and insects.

• Unplug from social media and use your free time to start a creative project, color, draw, paint, or read a book.

• Do some gardening. Watching things grow connects us directly with nature, while working in a garden teaches us patience, diligence, and attentiveness. A garden is a wonderful place to relax, reflect, and recharge your batteries.

IMPROVING THE ENVIRONMENT

We are inextricably connected to our planet—nature is our support system, and the way in which we treat the earth will have an impact on our future. So in looking at our spiritual wellbeing, we must also look to the wellbeing of our environment. Here are some ways in which we can improve it.

REDUCE, REUSE, AND RECYCLE

Plastic kills millions of sea birds and marine mammals and takes hundreds or even thousands of years to degrade, so the first thing you can do to improve the environment is reduce your use of plastic, especially single-use plastic. Use reusable shopping bags and avoid buying plastic bottles, cutlery, straws, and disposable cups. Choose eco-friendly cleaning products, cosmetics, clothing, and gift wrap. Volunteer for clean-ups in your community. You can also cut down on what you throw away by shopping wisely and then giving any unwanted clothes, household items, and toys to charity shops.

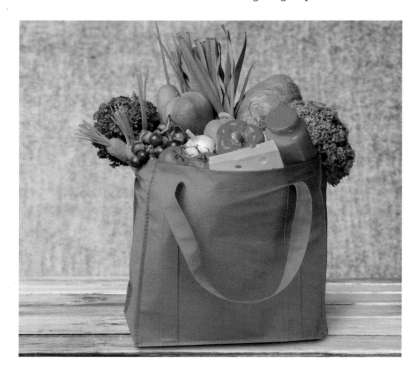
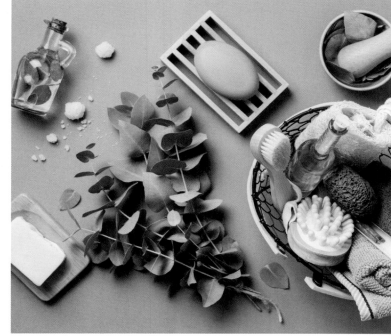

GROW PLANTS!

Planting things is not only an incredibly therapeutic activity in itself, but it also helps the environment in every way. Plants take in carbon dioxide and give out oxygen, so wherever there are plants, the air quality is better and the effects of pollution are reduced. Whether you choose a small houseplant, a pretty window box, a few flowers or a tree, growing plants is a rewarding way to improve our connection to nature and help the environment at the same time. Eco gardening, or "planet-friendly gardening," is the best way of all to look after our natural environment—use peat-free compost, plant the types of flowers that are suitable for insect pollinators, provide nest boxes, food and water for birds, and put up bamboo hotels for bees. This will increase the biodiversity in your garden and help your local wildlife to thrive.

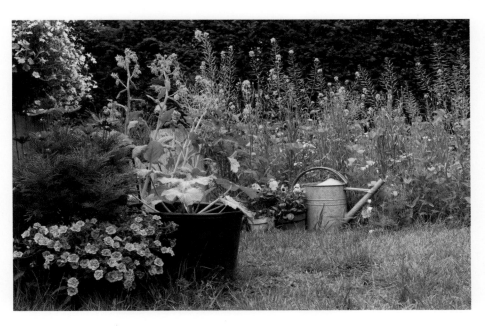

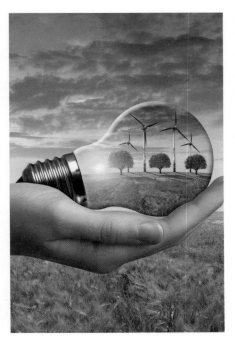

REDUCE YOUR CARBON FOOTPRINT

Your carbon footprint consists of the total amount of greenhouse gases (such as carbon dioxide and methane) that are generated by your actions. Greenhouse gases are released during the combustion of fossil fuels, such as coal, oil, and natural gas, to produce electricity. You can reduce your carbon footprint in the following ways:

- When traveling, leave the car at home and go by another method—walk or cycle for short distances, or use public transport for longer journeys. When going on holiday, consider a "staycation" instead of getting on a plane.
- Reduce the amount of electricity you use by buying energy-efficient lightbulbs, switching lights off when you leave a room, turning your TV off rather than leaving it on standy-by, unplugging chargers when your devices are fully charged, and using renewable energy sources such as solar power.
- Shop locally. This helps to cut carbon emissions and air pollution because what you buy will have fewer "food miles."
- Reduce your consumption of meat and dairy products. An article in the journal *Science* reported that the loss of wild areas to agriculture is the leading cause of the current mass extinction of wildlife. Further, it is believed that eating less meat and dairy would actually have a greater beneficial impact on our planet than any other single factor.

GIVE YOUR BRAIN A BOOST

Keep your brain in sharp and healthy with these quick-fix tips.

TOP UP ON OMEGAS
Eating a diet rich in omega-3 fatty acids, including DHA and EPA, is said to give your brain a powerful boost. DHA is the main player and forms the basis of omega fatty acids in your brain. It's essential for your central nervous system to function. The best source comes from oily fish such as sardines, salmon, and mackerel.

HYDRATE YOUR HEAD!
Your brain is more than 70 percent water, so it relies on you staying properly hydrated to function at its best.

MAXIMIZE YOUR SLEEP QUALITY
Snoozing, dozing, catching some Zs... whatever you call it, getting good-quality rest is essential for brain health. Sleep is when your brain can make sense of the day's activities and file away information.

CELEBRATE CELERY
Fill your plate with this crunchy green herb, as research by the University of Illinois found it contains luteolin, a compound that may help combat Alzheimer's disease and other degenerative mental illnesses. This is because luteolin reduces age-related inflammation in the brain and related memory loss by directly inhibiting the release of inflammatory molecules.

KEEP YOUR BRAIN HAPPY
Just like your body after a spot of over-indulgence, your brain also enjoys a detox from time to time to stay at its best. With this in mind, clinical hypnotherapist Fiona Lamb (fionalamb.com) has launched Mind Detox, which is designed to help you manage your mental health and organize your thoughts. The app boasts a host of tailored meditation sessions covering a range of topics from "mindfulness for worrying" to "mindpower healing."

SING THE PRAISES OF SINGING!

Do you enjoy belting out a tune in the shower or recreating your own carpool karaoke session in the rush hour? Then you're already helping your brain health without even realizing. Vocal coach Mark De-Lisser has been running community choirs for more than 15 years and has seen the physical and mental health benefits of singing, including boosted memory and concentration. "Singing uses the right side of the brain, which improves your ability to problem solve," explains Mark. "And when you memorize the lyrics to a new song, this stimulates the release of acetylcholine—the chemical responsible for your memory." So next time your favorite anthem comes on the radio, sing it loud and proud!

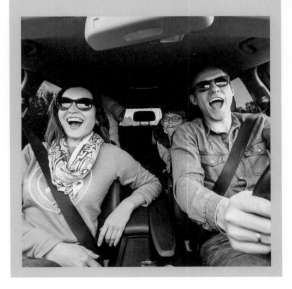

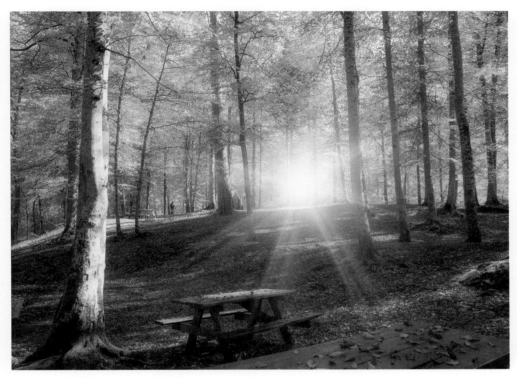

DOSE UP ON SUNSHINE

Lack of sun exposure can lead to low serotonin levels, which makes you more susceptible to depression, so try to get outside in daylight for at least half an hour a day.

BOOST B12

If you're embracing a mostly plant-based lifestyle, consider supplementing with B12, which is only found in meat and fish. The vitamin is thought to be responsible for preventing loss of neurons in your brain, and a deficiency is linked to memory loss and fatigue.

STAY ALERT WITH LEMON BALM

Improve your mental focus and perform well under pressure thanks to lemon balm leaf extract. It's been shown to regulate mood and emotion, as well as enhance memory, boost alertness and concentration, and also promote feelings of peace and tranquility.

HOW TO HALT MIGRAINES

If you ever get migraine headaches, there are some new—and ancient!—therapies that may help you find relief from your symptoms.

It is estimated that a whopping 15–20 percent of us suffer from migraines, making it the third most prevalent illness in the world, according to the World Health Organization. Migraines are thought to be a hereditary neurological condition caused by a particular genetic mutation. This mutation affects a particular protein that's designed to inhibit electrical activity in the brain. The intense pain is basically the brain getting irritated by something (whether hormones or an external trigger) and trying to slow things down. That's why the headaches are often accompanied by blurred vision and feelings of sickness, combined with confusion for the trigeminal nerve—the one that runs on both sides of your head and face, and which controls the muscles that make you chew. This nerve then sends out pain signals. In short, it's a miserable experience. But there are lots of new—and also old, tried and tested—treatments that can help.

STRETCH IT OUT

Yoga has various benefits that can reduce headaches—from relaxing tight muscles in your neck and jaw, to boosting blood flow to your brain. One study found that doing a yoga class five days a week for six weeks straight was able to reduce both the frequency and intensity of headaches and migraines.

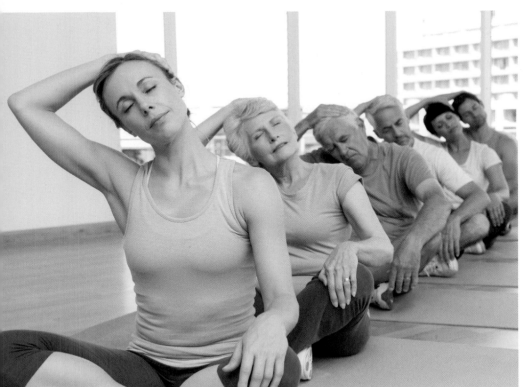

Left: This yoga exercise helps to stretch out your neck muscles. Place your hand on your head and very gently pull your right ear down toward your right shoulder. Pause while breathing in and out to a slow count of ten. Then do the same on the other side.

HEAD FOR A MASSAGE

As with yoga, massaging your neck, jaw, and scalp can help to boost circulation and relax your mind and body—all of which is conducive to reduced pain. "A monthly Indian head massage helps me," says Tahira Khan, 40. "I'd been getting menstrual migraines for the past 12 years after I had my daughter. I was prescribed Naproxen by the GP, but I hated taking tablets, so I decided to try Indian head massage. It's practiced in my Asian culture from when we're young and is a bonding experience between a mother and daughter. I've found if I get this done a week before my period, I don't get migraines. So, I exchange a monthly session with my mum, sisters, and daughter whenever possible."

TRY IT: Gently apply lavender massage oil to your temples, then sweep your fingers across your forehead along your hairline. Continue sweeping behind both ears and down toward your neck with slow, firm strokes.

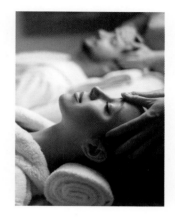

GET STRAIGHT TO THE POINT

There's good scientific evidence that acupuncture can help with headaches. "Acupuncture makes me feel brilliant," says Gill Lockhart, 62. "I was due to have acupuncture for my frozen shoulder but started getting a migraine about two hours before the appointment. I went anyway and told the acupuncturist, but she said the treatment would help that too. Afterwards I realized my migraine had gone."

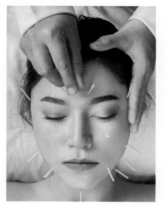

PULSE IT OUT

Many people swear by External Trigeminal Nerve Stimulation devices (e-TNS). These small machines can be used at home. You place an adhesive patch on your forehead for a short time, and it sends a current into your brain that is believed to interrupt the activity associated with a migraine. Studies have been encouraging: 85 percent of acute migraine sufferers trying the Cefaly device experienced pain relief. **Note:** It is recommended that you talk to your doctor before using a device such as this.

THINK AWAY THE PAIN

Neurolinguistic programming (NLP) is a method for working with your thought processes to change behaviors, but it is also believed to help with pain such as migraines. It's thought that using certain visualizations can help you tackle the problem without using medication, as well as reducing your stress levels.

TRY IT: NLP practitioner Rebecca Lockwood suggests you identify a color that in your mind relates to the pain. "Then imagine the color turning white. If the pain persists, repeat the process until the color turns and remains white," she says.

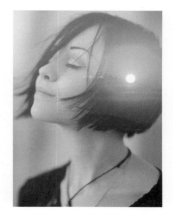

NATURAL BACK PAIN REMEDIES

The number of people affected by back pain at some point in their lives is shockingly high—the estimated figure in the UK and US is around 80 percent. These gentle tips and healing therapies will help you feel better.

HERBS AND OILS

Turning to nature could help nip back pain in the bud. "Some herbs have anti-inflammatory properties similar to non-steroidal anti-inflammatory drugs (NSAIDS)," says Dr. Dick Middleton, registered pharmacist and director of the British Herbal Medicine Association. Good examples of anti-inflammatory herbs are:

- Ginger (*Zingiber officinale*) rhizome.
- Turmeric (*Curcuma longa*) rhizome.
- Devil's claw (*Harpagophytum procumbens*) tuber.
- Licorice (*Glycyrrhiza glabra*) rhizome.
- European goldenrod (*Solidago virgaurea*).

As well as herbs, people have used essential oils as natural pain relievers for hundreds of years. The following relieve pain naturally, as well as promoting a sense of peace and relaxation:

- Lavender (*Lavandula angustifolia*) essential oil.
- Rosemary (*Rosmarinus officinalis*) essential oil.
- Peppermint (*Mentha piperita*) essential oil.
- Eucalyptus (*Eucalyptus*) essential oil.

DID YOU KNOW?

28.2 million... that's how many working days are lost each year in the UK due to musculoskeletal problems, including back, neck, and shoulder pain.

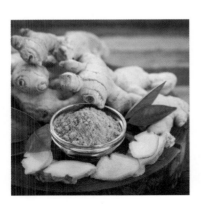
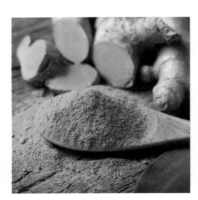
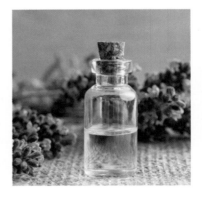
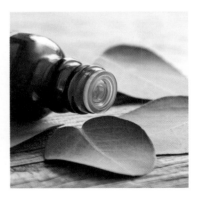

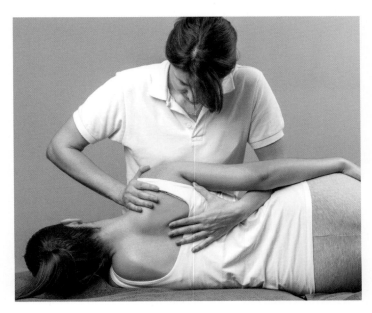

OSTEOPATHY

The principle underlying osteopathy is that our health and wellbeing depend on the smooth and cooperative fucntioning of our bones, muscles, ligaments, and connective tissues, and that if everything is correctly balanced, the body will heal itself. Osteopathy involves physical manipulation of the body's muscle tissue and bones, so an osteopath will move, stretch and massage your muscles and joints. The techniques aim to reduce pain, improve movement and encourage blood flow. Osteopathy is suitable for conditions such as:

- Lower back pain.
- Uncomplicated neck pain (as opposed to neck pain after an injury such as whiplash).
- Shoulder pain and elbow pain (such as tennis elbow, for example).
- Arthritis.
- Problems with the pelvis, hips, and legs.
- Sports injuries.
- Muscle and joint pain associated with driving, work, or pregnancy.

GET AN APP

The first medically approved app for back pain, Kaia (kaiahealth.com), is the largest musculoskeletal (MSK) platform worldwide. Its founders, Konstantin Mehl and Manuel Thurner, both suffered from years of back pain themselves, and then joined forces on a mission to find an effective way of managing chronic back pain and making it accessible to everyone—anytime, anywhere. Their digital platform is a clinically validated mind-body therapy that includes simple video exercises to relieve pain, and lets you chat online with physiotherapists to learn more about back health.

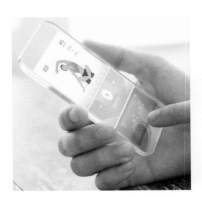
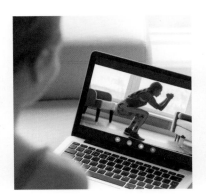
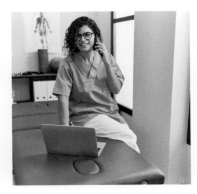
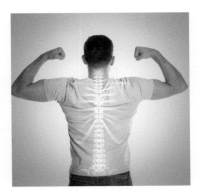

BEAT COLDS AND FLU

Eating homemade soup, wrapping up warm, and having a positive mindset can all help you stay well during the winter months.

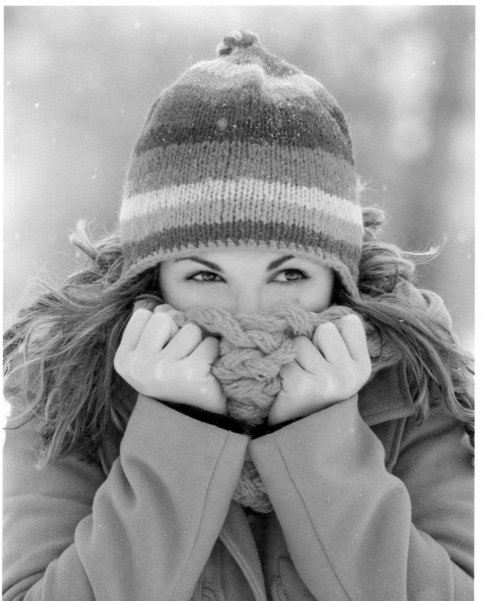

WRAP UP WARM

Feeling the chill? Staying warm could increase your chances of catching the common cold. A 2017 study by researchers at Mahidol University in Thailand found that chilled immune cells are less effective at fighting infection. However, simply cranking the central heating up high can dry out your skin, cause a scratchy throat, and even promote the spread of germs. Instead, layer up with cosy cardigans and blankets, and wrap up warm when outdoors.

COOK UP CHICKEN SOUP

This sickness staple isn't just an old wives' tale. "A hearty bowl of chicken and vegetable soup can slow the speed at which neutrophils move around your body," says nutritional therapist and health coach Ailsa Hichens (foodfabulous.co.uk). "Neutrophils are a type of white blood cell that protect your body from infection. When they move slowly, they're able to become more concentrated in areas that need them most, helping to fight infection."

TIP: Boil some bones and root veg for a few hours, simmering gently, then strain and have it for your main meal or sip throughout the day.

THE UPSIDE OF COLDS

Believe it or not, getting the occasional cold is actually a good thing—even though it may not feel like it as you tear into your fifth box of tissues! "It's a sign that your immune system is working normally and able to put up a good fight against invading viruses," says medical herbalist Hannah Charman (physichealth.uk). "It's a great opportunity for your body to cleanse itself of toxins and, if you're lucky, a chance to get some much needed rest."

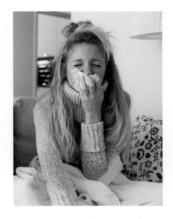

SOAK UP THE SALT

Salt crystals have been used for centuries to treat respiratory issues by cleansing the lungs so they better absorb oxygen, which helps boost immunity. Try the Cisca Easy Salt pipe, a natural dry salt inhaler that alleviates sneezing, coughing, and shortness of breath.

ONLINE HEALTH SUPPORT

An app might not be able to cure the common cold, but it can offer you some support. Home Remedies Plus (a free app) is a complete guide to creating remedies using common kitchen cupboard ingredients. Simply input your symptoms and the app will give you practical suggestions for what to do.

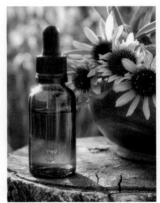

YOUR STEADFAST FLU FAVORITE

Echinacea is one of the most popular natural cold and flu remedies on the market, and it's easy to see why. The latest Swiss research has found that its antiviral and antibacterial properties actually prevent viruses and bacteria from clinging to respiratory tissues, dramatically reducing the risk of infection.

GET A HEALTHY DOSE OF VITAMIN D

Vitamin D is essential for strong immunity. It's particularly powerful at preventing upper respiratory tract infections, including rhinitis, tonsillitis, and laryngitis. Sunlight is the best way for your body to make this vitamin, but when the winter sun is too weak, you can top up naturally with vitamin D-rich foods such as oily fish, mushrooms, and eggs.

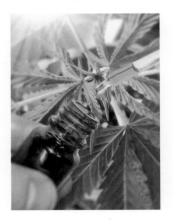

TRY A HERBAL HERO

Cannabidiol (CBD) oil may help with cold and flu symptoms. It's thought the cannabinoids and terpenes help reduce inflammation in your nose, throat, and lungs.

5 VIRUS-PREVENTION STRATEGIES

It's not a good idea to rely too much on antibiotics—as we build up resistance to them, they're less effective. So here are some other ways to help you fend off viruses.

1. Support your gut

With up to 70 percent of your immune cells located in your gut, and the bacteria there playing an essential role in supporting a strong immune system, it makes sense to support your good bugs. One way to do that is with fermented foods and/or probiotic supplements. "Taken over time, multi-strain probiotics (live bacterial supplements) have been shown to significantly shorten common colds and reduce the severity of symptoms," says Hannah Braye, nutritional therapist at Bio-Kult.

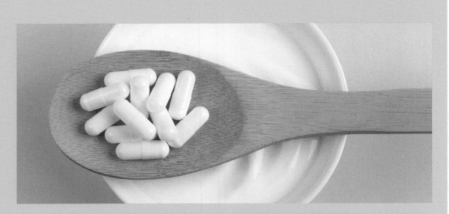

2. Look after your lungs

The COVID-19 virus obstructs respiratory pathways with thick mucus, which solidifies and blocks airways and lungs. However, the virus remains in your throat for 3–4 days before it gets to your lungs, so during that time you have a window of opportunity to kill it off with the following measures:

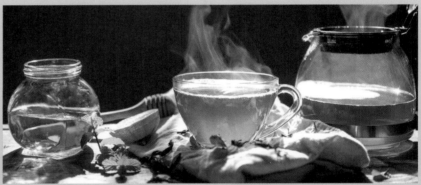

- Drink hot liquids. Coffee, tea, soups, and hot water all count. Avoid eating and drinking cold things.
- Gargle with an antiseptic. Add vinegar, salt, or lemon juice to warm water each day and gargle.
- Use a nebulizer. If you do catch a virus, you can prevent it from traveling down into your lungs by using a nebulizer with a 3 percent hydrogen peroxide solution (which is very weak), as recommended by Dr Thomas E. Levy, cardiologist and virus expert.

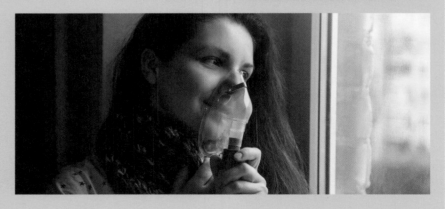

3. Supplement your vitamin D

As well as getting enough sunlight and eating foods that are rich in vitamin D (such as oily fish, mushrooms, and eggs), you can top up your vitamin D by taking a supplement. "Research shows that taking a vitamin D3 supplement can reduce the risk of getting a respiratory tract infection (including the common cold, influenza, and pneumonia) by a third compared with placebo," says Dr. Sarah Brewer. The benefits are even greater in people with an existing vitamin D deficiency. "There is also preliminary evidence published in the Irish Medical Journal that having a good vitamin D status may help to improve outcomes in people infected with the coronavirus. Although this is by no means certain, I recommend a dose of 25–50 mcg for adults, based on age—those over the age of 50 need a higher dose as their ability to synthesise vitamin D3 in the sun, and ability to absorb and use it, is reduced," she says.

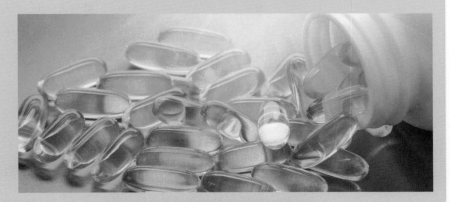

4. Don't rely on antibac

Antibacterial hand gels won't kill viruses; they only kill bacteria. Soap and water can reduce your chances of catching a virus by 21 percent if you always wash your hands well, but they also don't kill viruses. Try a colloidal silver spray such as Results RNA Extra Strength Silver, which does kill viruses.

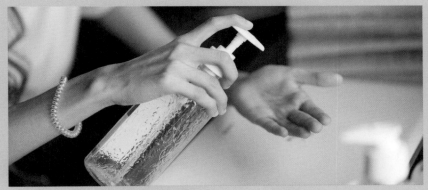

5. Get good sleep

Having a good 7–8 hours of uninterrupted rest really helps your immune system stay strong. Feeling relaxed before bed helps, so try a magnesium supplement plus a relaxing pillow spray.

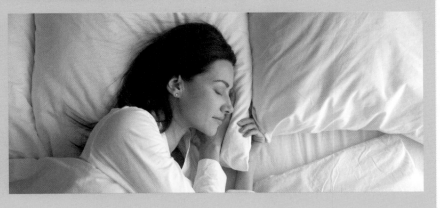

12 TWEAKS TO BEAT TYPE 2 DIABETES

Type 2 diabetes is a condition that causes the level of sugar (glucose) in the blood to become too high. It can be linked to being overweight, inactive, or having a history of it in the family, but making certain lifestyle changes can keep it in check and even reverse it altogether.

The two main type of diabetes are called type 1 and type 2. The former is where the body can't make any insulin at all (the hormone that allows your body to use glucose for energy), so insulin injections are required for life, but the vast majority of diabetic people have type 2. Symptoms include excessive thirst, needing to urinate frequently, and fatigue, and it can increase the risk of serious problems with eyes, heart, and nerves. But the good news is that by adopting a healthy lifestyle and diet, you can improve your blood sugar balance. Here are 12 ways to beat type 2 diabetes:

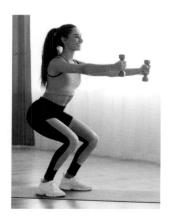

1. PUMP THOSE WEIGHTS!

Weight training improves your body's ability to process sugar, which in turn reduces your chances of getting diabetes—or improving the condition if you already have it. Basically, the more lean muscle mass you have, the easier it is for insulin to move sugar out of your blood and into your muscles, where it's needed. This is because muscle cells house insulin receptors, and the more muscle, the more insulin receptors you have. Equally, if you exercise your largest muscles (i.e. the ones in your legs and bottom) before you eat something sugary, it helps prime your body to better absorb the sugar. So, when you're squatting or doing a deadlift in the gym, you're not only toning your body, but helping it process sugar!
Blood sugar balancer: Do 30 squats before you eat your main meal.

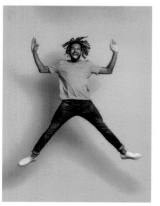

2. HYPE UP THE HIIT

High Intensity Interval Training (HIIT) is an effective way to build lean muscle mass, lose weight, and improve insulin sensitivity. HIIT can be performed in various ways, for example jogging on the spot for 30 seconds flat out, followed by 30 seconds of star jumps, 30 seconds of vertical jumps, and a rest for 30 seconds. Repeat the sequence 3–4 times.
Blood sugar balancer: If you are new to exercise, start slowly—only do one round of a circuit, then build up week by week.

3. STEP TO IT

Although weight training and HIIT are the most effective physical ways of improving insulin sensitivity, increasing your daily steps will still help.

Blood sugar balancer: Aim to walk 6,000–10,000 steps per day.

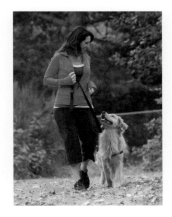

4. SLEEP ON IT

Sleep is crucial for mental and physical repair. Poor sleep leads to increased cortisol, which tells your body you're in flight-or-fight mode, leading to increased glycogen in your blood. This will make you crave sweet things to replace the glycogen you have used up. Added to this, lack of sleep also instructs your body to increase the hormone ghrelin, which tells you to eat more!

Blood sugar balancer: If your sleep is poor, try a magnesium supplement before bed to help you relax. Look for magnesium threonate (a salt of magnesium combined with L-Threonate), which has been proven by studies at MIT in the US to help reduce anxiety and improve sleep quality.

5. CURB YOUR CORTISOL

High levels of cortisol, the hormone secreted when you're under chronic or acute stress, can lead to high blood sugar. This is because when you're under stress, your body's need for glucose increases. Cortisol is secreted as an "emergency response" to trigger the release of glycogen, which is your body's stored sugar. Having too much glycogen coursing through your veins is damaging if it's not utilized by your muscles, which it would normally be if you were in a real fight-or-flight situation. So it's not just what you eat that affects your blood sugar—your stress level affects it too, which is why making time for relaxation is so important.

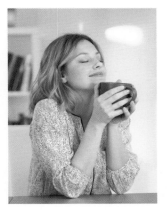

Blood sugar balancer: Upon waking, do 10 long, slow, deep breaths to start your day in a calm way. Do these whenever you feel stressed throughout the day.

6. FIGHT BACK WITH FATS

Good polyunsaturated fats such as those in avocados, olives, nuts, and oily fish help to stabilize blood sugar. Fats provide energy and help you to absorb nutrients and manufacture hormones. A study at Cambridge University found that consuming good fats lowered people's risk of getting diabetes compared with consuming certain carbohydrates.

Blood sugar balancer: Drizzle walnut oil on salads, as it is rich in omega oils.

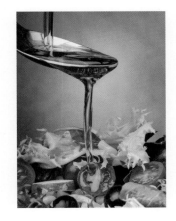

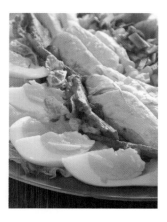

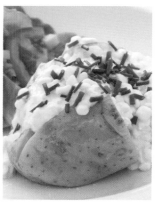

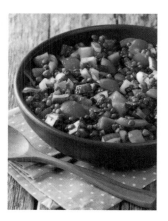

7. POWER UP WITH PROTEIN

Protein-rich foods such as chicken, beef, turkey, and eggs help your body to detoxify, relax, and maintain stable blood sugar levels. This is because your system has to break them down to process them, so they don't end up as instant sugar—unlike protein shakes. Liquid protein raises your blood sugar, as it doesn't need much breaking down by your digestive system (the same goes for some so-called "healthy" juices—these have the blood-sugar-raising effect on your body that you'd get from drinking cola).
Blood sugar balancer: Eat most of your protein first during your meal, as this will slow down the absorption of any carbohydrates you consume.

8. ADD LEMON AND VINEGAR

Squeezing lemon juice or drizzling vinegar over vegetables reduces the effect of the food on blood sugar. Both are acidic, and this helps slow the rate of digestion and the rate at which your stomach empties, giving the added benefit of making you feel fuller for longer.
Blood sugar balancer: Make a simple salad dressing with ½ cup olive oil, ¼ cup cider vinegar, 3 tbsp fresh lemon juice, ½ tsp salt, ¼ tsp black pepper, and 1 clove of crushed garlic.

9. FEAST ON FERMENTED FOODS

Regularly eating fermented foods such as yogurt, cottage cheese, sauerkraut, or kefir reduces your risk of diabetes by an incredible 24 percent. This was found in a study by the medical research unit at Cambridge University, involving 25,000 people over an 11-year period.
Blood sugar balancer: Top a baked potato with plenty of butter and a dollop of cottage cheese. The fats and protein will reduce how quickly your body will absorb the carbs in the potato.

10. SWEETEN WITH STEVIA

Try the herb stevia. It can give you that sweet hit without rapidly raising your blood sugar like table sugar does. Another alternative is xylitol, a sugar alcohol made from birch trees, or a plant called xylan. Similar to stevia, xylitol is sweet but doesn't significantly raise your insulin level.
Blood sugar balancer: Try Total Sweet 100% Natural Xylitol Sugar Alternative from a health food shop.

11. FILL UP WITH FIBER

A recent survey by Ryvita found that 42 percent of Brits don't eat a single piece of fiber-rich fruit or veg each day. Fiber not only reduces your risk of type 2 diabetes, but also cuts down your chances of developing bowel cancer, strokes, and heart disease. It keeps your intestines healthy and also slows down the rate at which food is converted into sugar and then absorbed into your bloodstream, thereby helping maintain stable blood sugar. Soluble fiber includes pectins, found in fruit, and beta glucans, found in oats. Insoluble fiber is found in wholegrains and legumes. But whether it's the soluble kind or not, it's good to aim for 30 g (1 oz) of fiber per day.

Blood sugar balancer: Add lentils, chickpeas, or beans to your salads and stews.

12. SUPPORT WITH SUPPLEMENTS

Various supplements and herbs can help you manage your blood sugar by increasing insulin sensitivity. These include chromium, cinnamon, magnesium, fish oils, fenugreek, and gymnema leaf. Chromium, for example, activates an enzyme called tyrosine kinases, which allows insulin to better attach to receptor sites in cells, thereby improving sensitivity.

Blood sugar balancer: Things to try include adding cinnamon to porridge and taking a high-quality fish oil capsule daily. You could also take a fish oil such as Nordic Naturals Omega 3-D.

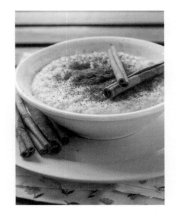

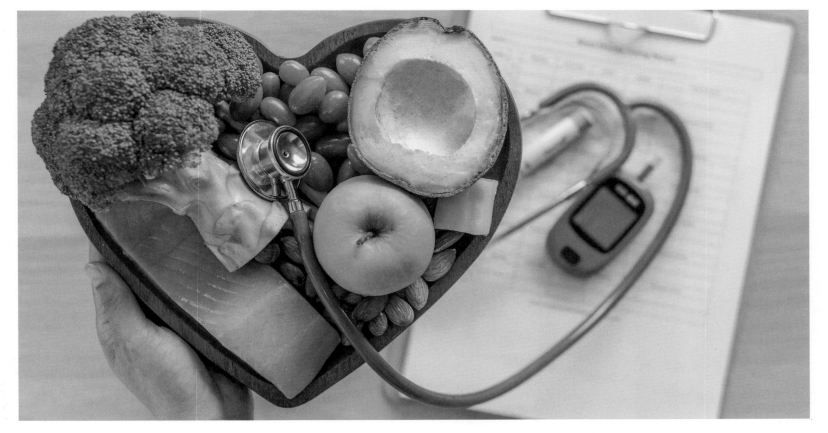

WOMEN'S HEALTH

Let's now turn to women's health and have a look at some of the issues that affect women's health and wellbeing.

REPRODUCTIVE AND SEXUAL HEALTH

Although women generally live longer than men, they face unique health risks in the areas of pregnancy and childbirth, with maternal mortality accounting for more that a quarter of a million deaths per year in first-world countries, and substantially greater numbers in the developing world. Here's a summary of female reproductive and sexual health issues:

- Pre-menstrual tension (PMS) and menstruation.
- Sex and gynaecological issues: includes painful sex, sexually transmitted infections such as HIV and AIDS, pelvic inflammatory disease, and female genital mutilation (FGM).
- Fertility, endometriosis, contraception, pregnancy, preeclampsia, abortion, miscarriage, childbirth, and breastfeeding.
- Menopause.

OTHER HEALTH ISSUES FOR WOMEN

Of course women face many other health issues too, with cardiovascular disease being the leading cause of death in women worldwide, accounting for one-third of all female deaths. Here are some of the many health issues that women may face:

- Heart disease, high blood pressure, stroke, and chronic obstructive pulmonary disease (COPD).
- Cancers, such as breast, ovarian, and cervical cancer.
- Depression and anxiety, including post-natal depression and concerns about body image.
- Domestic violence, abuse, and issues realting to sexual consent.
- Gender equality.
- Autoimmune diseases, including sclerosis, rheumatoid arthritis, psoriasis, and celiac disease.
- Osteoporosis.
- Dementia.

DID YOU KNOW?

"Cardiovascular disease kills more women than men, and even in women aged less than 65 years, more than twice as many women die of cardiovascular diseases than of breast cancer."
Prof. Hugo Katus, Advocacy Committee Chair, European Society of Cardiology

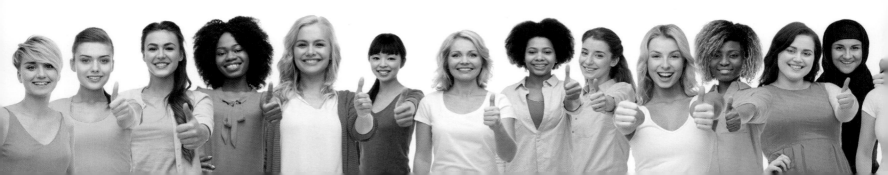

WELLNESS TIPS
FOR WOMEN

Here are some useful reminders for how women can keep healthy, energized, and ready to deal with whatever life thows their way.

• Choose natural foods; don't skip meals and try to limit your intake of salt, sugar, caffeine and alcohol. Keep well hydrated—drink about 6–8 glasses of water per day, or more if you're exercising or the weather is warm.

• Exercise regularly to keep fit. Aim for at least 30 minutes of movement four days a week. Cardio exercise is best, which includes walking, running, dancing, and swimming. Also do some stretching exercise such as yoga or Pilates—and don't forget your pelvic floor exercises, too!

• Control stress and anxiety with meditation. Take time out when you need to, and prioritize your mental health needs.

• If you have any specific concerns, research them. For example, certain foods and exercises should be avoided during pregnancy. Talk to friends, read books, and go online to learn more about your particular stage in life.

• Consult with your doctor and dentist every year, and keep all your appointments for mammograms and smear tests. If you notice anything unusual—from a new spot on your skin to a change in the condition of your hair—go and see your doctor.

• Stick to a bedtime routine and make sure you get enough sleep.

MEN'S HEALTH

While men don't have the same reproductive and sexual problems as women, they do have their own health issues, and unfortunately many men still find it difficult to talk about their problems or go to the doctor.

The stereotypical idea that men are strong or don't cry has had a huge negative effect in Western society—unfortunately some men skip their regular medical check-ups and don't ask for help when they need it. And not taking their physical and mental health seriously means that men can develop serious health problems later on. As it is, men tend to die about five years earlier than women, so the "medical gender gap" is very real.

"A healthy attitude is contagious but don't wait to catch it from others. Be a carrier."
Tom Stoppard

HEALTH ISSUES FOR MEN

Like women, more men die of heart disease than any other cause of death, with cancer being the second leading cause of death. Here's a summary of some male health issues:

- Heart disease, high blood pressure, stroke, and chronic obstructive pulmonary disease (COPD).
- Cancers, such as prostate, testicular, bowel, and bladder cancer, and human papillomavirus (HPV) which can cause cancer.
- Depression and anxiety.
- Suicide—men are three times more likely than women to commit suicide.
- Sexual problems, such as erectile dysfuntion and low testosterone.
- COVID-19—men and women have the same prevalence, but men are more at risk for worse outcomes and death, independent of age.
- Alcoholism, liver disease, gout, kidney stones, and duodenal ulcers.
- Diabetes.
- Emphysema.
- Hemophilia.
- Unintentional injuries.

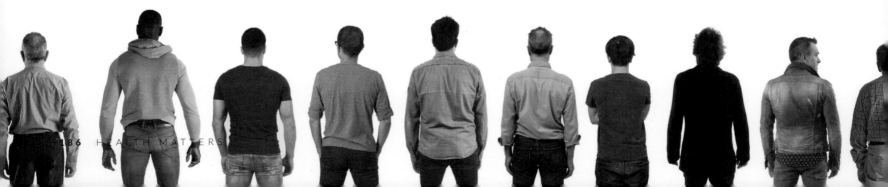

WELLNESS
TIPS FOR MEN

The good news is that men can do a lot to take control of their health, starting with prioritizing prevention. Here are some steps men can take to avoid common health problems at any age:

• Eat a healthy diet and drink about 6–8 glasses of water per day. Try to limit your intake of salt, sugar, and caffeine, and if you choose to drink alcohol, drink it in moderation.

• Manage your weight by getting more exercise. Men tend to have more belly fat than women, but losing a few pounds will lower your risk of cardiovascular disease, diabetes, and certain cancers, not to mention increasing health and happiness.

• Give up smoking. Use aids to help you, and keep cravings at bay by staying busy.

• Be more emotionally vulnerable and don't be afraid to talk to someone or seek help if you're feeling down. Note that men sometimes experience depression as anger or irritability rather than sadness. Don't sweep these feelings under the rug—talk to a friend, partner, or health professional.

• See your doctor and dentist every year, and when you're invited to cancer screening tests, go straight away without procrastinating!

• Go to bed at the same time every night and turn off your phone, tablet, and computer at least an hour before bedtime. Give yourself plenty of time to relax and unwind.

BECOMING A PARENT

The day you become a parent is life-changing and hopefully the start of a hugely rewarding experience, but when you haven't slept for days and your baby is crying at 4 o'clock in the morning, you might need some help. Here are a few suggestions and strategies:

GREAT EXPECTATIONS

There are bound to be mixed emotions when a baby comes along. On one hand your hopes and dreams may have come true, but on the other hand you might feel overwhelmed at the enormity of the challenges ahead and your endless new responsibilities. For some, their sense of self can be considerably eroded as they no longer feel like the person they used to be—they are now a "parent," with financial, emotional, and care-giving responsibilites and a completely new identity. These feelings are entirely natural and normal, and all part of the process of becoming a parent. Here are a few important reminders:

- Be realistic and kind to yourself.
- Eat healthily and get some sleep whenever you can.
- There's no "right" or "wrong" way of doing things, so don't beat yourself up if your reality doesn't match up to your expectations. Try not to catastrophize.
- Remember that you have your own intrinsic value, no matter what is going on with your child.

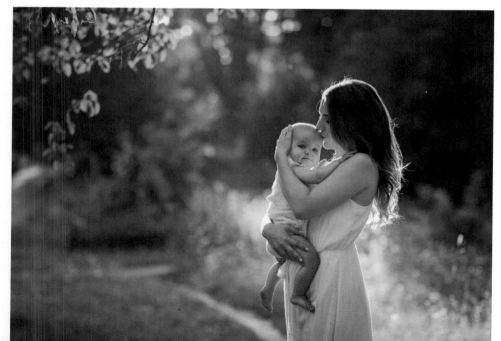

TAKE TIME TO ADJUST

It goes without saying that as a new parent, you've recently been through a miraculous—and possibly traumatic—physical and emotional experience. New mothers will undergo major changes to their bodies: "You've probably got a flabby tummy, stretchmarks, your nipples might be sore, your perineum might be sore, you might have back pain, you might be leaking milk, you might have piles, you might be experiencing leaking and discharge," says Maggie Fisher, a specialist health visitor and Professional Development Officer at the Institute of Health Visiting. So it's important to give yourself time to heal and to adjust to your new body.

New fathers also go through a major transformative experience and need time to adjust. They might benefit from the following suggestions:

- Do some research about parenthood and decide on the father you would like to be.
- Keep as physically fit and healthy as possible.
- Talk about parenting with your co-parent and keep the channels of communication open at all times.
- Find fellow fathers in your local area and exchange ideas.
- Acknowledge and accept that your sex life may change.

Of course, there are many variations on the above—adoption, surrogacy, single-parent families, step-children, grandparent families, and same-sex parenting to name a few—but the principles remain the same. Every new parent or guardian faces major changes and challenges when raising a child, and it always takes time to adjust.

ASK FOR SUPPORT

Especially in the early days, it's completely normal for new parents to need a little extra support. This might involve having someone come over to wash the dishes, do the laundry, watch the baby while you get some sleep, or just provide a friendly face to give you some emotional support. Single parents in particular can benefit enormously from cultivating a good social network—friends, other parents, neighbors, and relatives—who can help with the new baby. So, have a think about what you need and then ask for support. Looking after your new baby during its first year is a constant and demanding job, but you don't have to go through it alone.

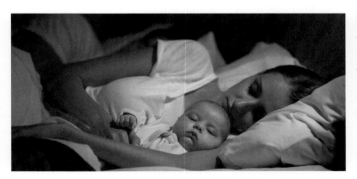

Note: If you don't feel connected to your baby after a few weeks or if you experience a high level of distress that begins to affect your ability to function, make an appointment to see a health professional. They are there to help you.

"Trust yourself. You know more than you think you do."
Benjamin Spock, pediatrician

6 REASONS WHY SLEEP MATTERS

Let's now turn to the subject of sleep. Getting a good night's sleep is not just vital for giving us energy, it is also crucial to our health and wellbeing.

Most of us don't get enough sleep. Research by the Mental Health Foundation shows one-third of us experience insomnia—and according to the Economic and Social Research Council, one in 10 of us now regularly takes medication to help us sleep. But lack of sleep doesn't just cause a frayed temper and red eyes—it also affects your health. Here's why solid shut-eye really counts.

1. IT REALLY IS BEAUTY SLEEP

You've probably noticed your skin looks fresher and brighter when you go to bed early. A study from University Hospitals Case Medical Center in Cleveland, Ohio, found that women who sleep well age better, and their skin recovers more quickly when it's put under stress factors such as sun exposure. Plus, poor sleepers have more signs of skin aging, including wrinkles, sagging, and pigmentation.

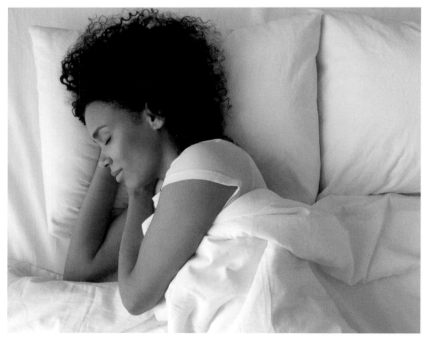

2. IT KEEPS YOUR MIND SHARP

Getting good-quality sleep can help lower your risk of dementia, according to US research. The scientists believe that during sleep your brain gets "cleaned"—and substances called beta-amyloid plaques, linked with Alzheimer's disease, are cleared away. If you miss out on sleep, there's an increased risk of plaques building up.

3. IT MAY REDUCE CANCER RISK

Some research is showing a link between poor sleep and some common forms of cancer. One study found sleeping for less than six hours a night puts you at a 50 percent increased risk of bowel cancer. Other research has linked lack of sleep with more aggressive breast cancer. Doctors believe that poor sleep disturbs your immune system and can trigger dangerous inflammation inside your body. And it maybe that the hormone melatonin, produced when you sleep, could help prevent cell damage that can lead to cancer.

4. IT BOOSTS YOUR IMMUNE SYSTEM

Studies on shift workers reveal a great deal about how lack of sleep damages the body's immune system. Daylight, which triggers wakefulness, is a stronger influence than even a deep need for sleep, so most shift workers average only five to five-and-a-half hours of sleep. If you constantly override your body clock's signals, you create a lot of stress in your body, which can dampen immunity. A study from the American Academy of Sleep Medicine found that sleeplessness causes a spike in white blood cells in a bid to boost immunity, which is the same way your body reacts to high stress. A recent study found that sleep helps to strengthen your immune system's memory—so you're better able to remember bugs you've come across before and mount a more effective defence against them.

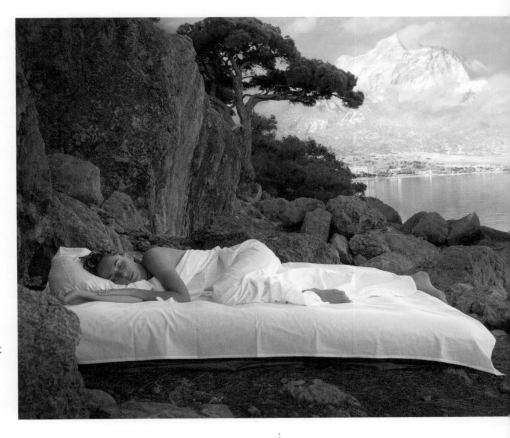

5. IT KEEPS YOU SLIM

People who sleep badly are more likely to be overweight. A study from the University of Stanford, in the US, found that poor sleep led to raised levels of ghrelin, a hormone that makes you feel hungry, and lower levels of leptin, another hormone linked with feelings of satiety (feeling full). That's why you may have found that you eat more after a bad night's sleep. So if you get enough sleep, you'll have much more control over the amount you eat.

6. IT CUTS YOUR RISK OF HEART DISEASE

If you regularly wake up feeling unrested due to poor sleep, you have a 63 percent higher risk of cardiovascular disease, according to research. A study by the American Heart Association found that sleeping for fewer than six hours a night increases inflammatory substances in the blood by 25 percent, raises blood pressure and heart rate, and affects blood sugar levels, which can raise your risk of heart disease and type 2 diabetes. Sufficient sleep will lower your risk.

HOW TO IMPROVE YOUR SLEEP

Getting adequate rest is essential for your health and wellbeing, but just how do you achieve more shut-eye? Read on for our good sleep guide...

We're all advised to get eight hours of sleep a night, but do we all manage it? We're all busy these days, so doesn't it make sense to stay up late or rise early to squeeze in a few extra tasks? We'd never get everything done otherwise. Actually, it does matter! During sleep, our body repairs itself and recovers from the rigors of the day. It's also the time when our mind processes everything that's happened during the day—making sense of it and learning lessons. If we sleep well, each day feels like a new beginning and a fresh start. Without good sleep, however, life can feel like one long uphill struggle.

WHILE YOU WEREN'T SLEEPING...

A lack of sleep—or the inability to achieve good-quality sleep—causes the body to produce extra adrenaline to keep us going, in an attempt to combat the tiredness. And this increased dependence on stress hormones places great demands on our system. In one study, published by *Science Daily*, it was found that people who began sleeping less than six to eight hours a night were subject to an accelerated cognitive decline, equivalent to four to seven years of aging. Other studies have found that poor sleep may speed up the onset, or increase the severity, of age-related conditions, such as type 2 diabetes, high blood pressure, obesity, and memory loss. In these studies, subjects also displayed lower levels of thyroid-stimulating hormones, which can lead to a slower metabolism. Lack of sleep also changes the hormone balance within the body, slowing the release of leptin into our system. Leptin is the hormone that signals the state of fat stores. Less of it means we don't appreciate when fat stores

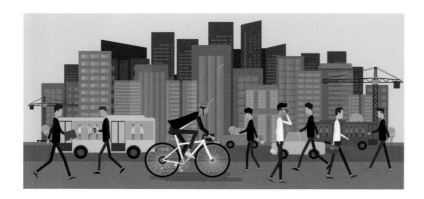

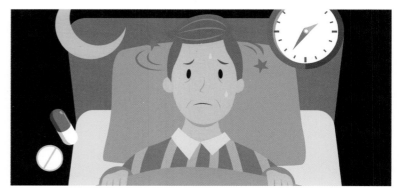

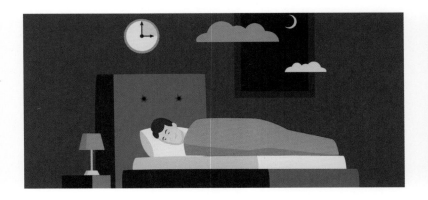
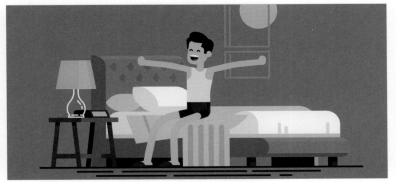

are full and so seek out more food. At the same time, sleep deprivation causes our body to release more ghrelin, the hormone that signals hunger. The most alarming aspect of many of the studies carried out on sleep is that just one week of sleep deprivation can be enough to disrupt the balance of the body and result in any of the above symptoms. We also don't need to lose a great deal of sleep for the consequences to be severe. One recent study suggested that just 30 minutes of sleep deprivation can increase the risk of obesity.

QUANTITY AND QUALITY

Good sleep is made up of two elements—quantity and quality. To optimize both, it's important that we get familiar with how much sleep we need. The majority of people manage on six to eight hours a night, but some can prosper on less, while others need more. If you're not sure how much sleep you need, the easiest way to find out is to experiment until you work it out. Most of us have a pretty consistent wake-up time, based around work or family, so adjust your bedtime, test out a few options over the course of a couple of weeks and see which one leaves you feeling most refreshed.

Once you know how much sleep you need, the advice is simple. It's all about routine. Ideally, we should maintain the same bedtime and wake-up time seven days a week. This isn't practical for most people, but the more we shift these times, the less likely we are to benefit from the best-quality sleep. If you struggle to fall asleep, this is often due to the fact you've packed so much into the day that you're running around right up until it's time to sleep. If this happens, you're unlikely to fall asleep quickly – it's difficult to go from operating at full speed to instantly achieving the relaxed state required for sleep. And even if you do fall asleep right away, there's a danger that you'll wake in the night as your mind attempts to deal with all the stimulation it has been subjected to up until the end of the day.

As well as determining your best bedtime, it helps to establish a pre-sleep routine. Many people think of pre-sleep as the last 10–20 minutes of the day, but ideally your pre-sleep routine should

"Innocent sleep. Sleep that soothes away all our worries. Sleep that puts each day to rest. Sleep that relieves the weary laborer and heals hurt minds. Sleep, the main course in life's feast, and the most nourishing."
William Shakespeare,
Macbeth

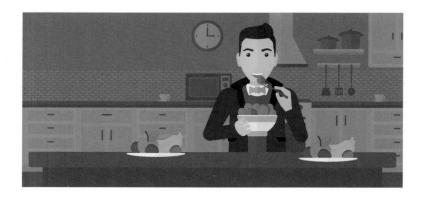

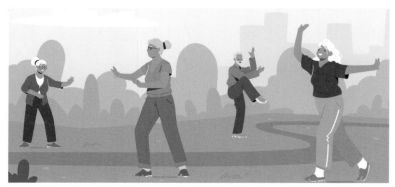

extend through the entire day. After all, everything we do while we're awake has a possible positive or negative effect on our sleep. For the best night-time recovery, think about everything you eat and drink through the day, in relation to your sleep routine. Too much caffeine, alcohol, sugary meals, snacks, and processed foods can all stimulate the system, playing havoc with blood sugar levels, making it hard to unwind in the evenings and have a good-quality night of rest. You should also give some thought to your activity routine. Exercise is a great way to manage your state of mind through the day, keep you calm and burn off any excess energy that could keep you awake at night.

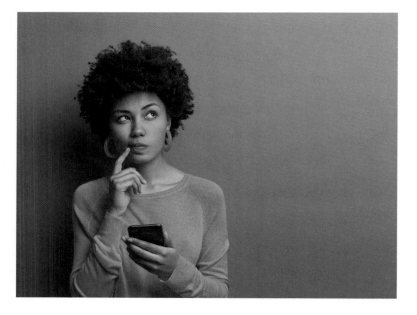

PLAYING ON REPEAT

Many people are kept awake at night by thoughts of the relationships they have with people during the day. This might be interaction with work colleagues, friends, family, your partner, or your children. Often thoughts of things we've done or said will play on our minds. There are a couple of things you can do to prevent this happening:

- Plan all your contact with other people. Be proactive rather than reactive, think about how you'd like all conversations to end, and approach them with this in mind.
- Plan some small breaks periodically throughout your day, during which you can review events so far. Think about what went well and make some notes on what you'd do differently in the future. Dealing with your day as it unfolds is a great way to avoid trying to process everything you've been through over the entire day just before you'd like to fall asleep.

- Look at is the pattern of your sleep cycles and whether you are a night owl or an early bird (see below). We all have sleep cycles, which last roughly 90–100 minutes, and for the best night's sleep it's important to maintain the integrity of these sleep cycles. So, for example, if you have 90-minute sleep cycles, seven-and-a-half hours of sleep would be five sleep cycles and you'd wake up feeling refreshed. This is why the consistency of your bedtime and wake-up time is so important—if you mistime your routine and wake up in the middle of the deep-sleep segment of a cycle, you'll feel groggy, find it difficult to get going and won't benefit from your rest as much as you would if you had completed full sleep cycles.

NIGHT OWL OR EARLY BIRD?

When planning your bedtime and wake time to cater for complete sleep cycles, you must take into account your preference for morning or night-time. Night owls will typically stay up later than early birds, but if you are a night owl, try not to stay up too late. Given that most people need to get up for work, it pays to not be fooling around at 3 am. Unfortunately, the world may not allow you to follow your ideal sleep routine—extreme night owls can struggle with the modern standard of a nine-to-five day, but with clear and consistent daytime, evening and pre-sleep routines, it's possible to make the most of the quantity and quality of sleep that you get.

GOOD NIGHT, SLEEP TIGHT

Is there an optimum window of time to be asleep? It has been demonstrated that between 11 pm and 1 am, adrenal glands recover and the gall bladder dumps toxins from the system. If you're asleep while all this is happening, these processes—along with other elements of recovery—can be more efficient. However, if you're not naturally asleep by 11 pm, the stress involved in trying to get to sleep to help your body recover can actually do more harm than good. For long-term sleep success, it's important to establish the routine that works best for you, enabling you to get everything done and allowing sufficient time for rest and recovery. There's a balance to be struck: if you get it right, you'll feel energized through the day, achieve a focused state of mind at all times, enjoy life and sleep well—all of which will limit any unnecessary signs of aging.

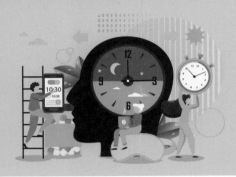

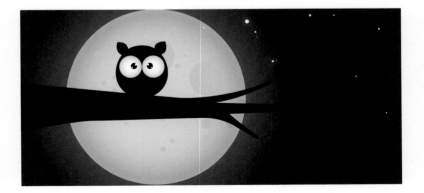

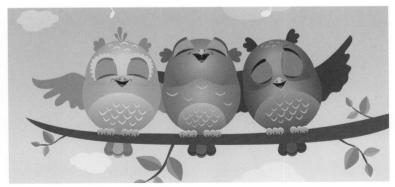

BEDTIME TIPS

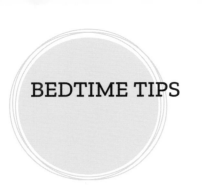

When it's time to wind down and get ready for bed, there are several practical things you can do to increase your chances of falling asleep.

LIGHT AND DARK

Our body has a natural time-keeping clock known as circadian rhythm. This tells us when to be awake and when to be asleep, and it's linked to our exposure to light. Natural sunlight or bright light during the day signals to our body that we should be awake, while at night our bodies release a hormone called melatonin to put us to sleep—but this only happens after we've been exposed to light during the day. So one of the best ways of ensuring a good night's sleep is to spend time outdoors during the day—even if only for a walk at lunchtime—and then make sure your bedroom is quiet and dark at bedtime. Switch off your television, computer and phone about an hour before you go to bed. Unfortunately, watching your favorite boxset, checking your social media, or reading an eBook on your iPad are among the worst things you can do just before bedtime. The blue light emitted from these electronic devices prevents the right amount of melatonin from being released and disrupts your sleep cycle.

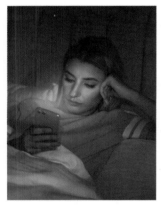

FOODS

It's best to avoid large meals before bedtime—these cause the body to focus on digestion rather than sleep. Try a lighter snack instead, ideally one containing tryptophan (an amino acid which increases the production of melatonin). Examples include a bowl of cereal, crackers and cheese, or toast with peanut butter (and see table opposite for some other snoozy foods). Avoid caffeine and alcohol—caffeine overactivates the mind, and alcohol stops you from entering the deep phase of your sleep cycle.

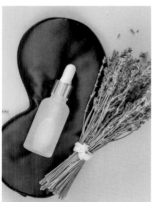

BEDROOM ENVIRONMENT

As well as keeping your bedroom dark, make sure it's the right temperature for sleep. This is ideally quite cool—around 15.5–19.5°C (60–67°F). Our bodies cool down as we fall asleep, so a cooler environment helps us to do this. You might try using a calming scent such as lavender, valerian, sweet marjoram, jasmine, lemon, or bergamot, or play some soothing music or a natural background sound such as rainfall or white noise. Choose a supportive mattress and wear natural, breathable fibres.

DEEP BREATHING

Try a mindfulness exercise or some deep breathing when you're ready to go to sleep. These help to slow your heart rate, reduce your blood pressure, and relieve anxiety and stress.

6 SNOOZY FOODS FOR BETTER SLEEP

1. ALMONDS are a natural source of melatonin and the sleep-promoting mineral magnesium, both of which can help you sleep more soundly. Try eating around 10 almonds before retiring or, if you prefer, drink a glass of almond milk.

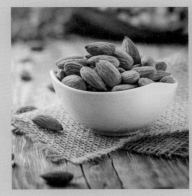

2. KIWI FRUIT are rich in serotonin and antioxidants, both of which may improve sleep quality. Research from Taipei Medical University found that volunteers eating two kiwi fruits before bed for four weeks fell asleep more quickly and slept more deeply and for longer.

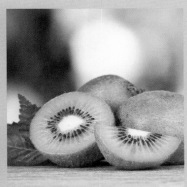

3. CHAMOMILE TEA is a popular choice before bedtime thanks to the calming effects of its antioxidant apigenin, which binds to specific receptors in the brain. This helps to decrease anxiety and initiate sleep.

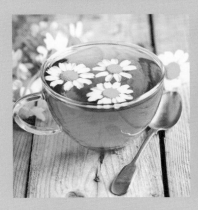

4. MONTMORENCY CHERRY JUICE is a natural source of melatonin, the hormone that regulates sleep. A study at Northumbria University showed that when participants drank two 30 ml (6 tsp) concentrated shots of cherry juice twice a day for a week, they slept 39 minutes longer, their sleep quality was better, and they felt less sleepy during the day.

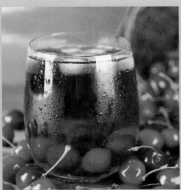

5. LETTUCE contains lactucarium (a milky fluid) that is a natural sedative. To make a sleep-inducing drink, blend the juice of one bag of fresh, organic lettuce with a banana (which is a good source of tryptophan), and some almond milk.

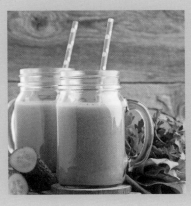

6. OATS are packed with soothing nutrients such as B vitamins and magnesium, which benefit your nervous system and can help alleviate anxiety. They are also a good vegetarian source of tryptophan. To help you feel calmer before bedtime, drink some oat milk or eat a small bowl of oatmeal.

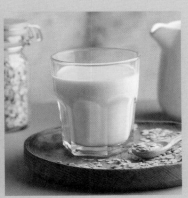

SLEEPY SCENTS

Lavender is always touted as being the smell to help you snooze, but there are plenty of other fragrances to get you into the sleep zone.

SANDALWOOD

The woody, sweet, aromatic scent of sandalwood is burned in Hindu and Buddhist temples. "The scent instils a sense of peace and tranquillity," says Jo Kellett, aromatherapist at Tissera Nd. "It's very relaxing, alleviates anxiety and eases mental fatigue. It's also restorative and emotionally grounding. If you're having problems sleeping, sandalwood will help you to switch off from the stresses of the day. Studies have shown that it contains components (santanols) that have a naturally sedative effect."

JASMINE

The sweet, heady scent of jasmine is as calming as Valium but with none of the side effects, as reported in the *Journal of Biological Chemistry*. Researchers at the Heinrich Heine University, Dusseldorf, found that the scent of this delicate white flower has the same calming, sedative effect on the central nervous system as commonly prescribed sleeping pills and sedatives. Brain scans showed that inhaling jasmine molecules enhanced the effect of gamma-aminobutyric acid (GABA)—an amino acid produced naturally in your brain—by more than five times. GABA promotes relaxation, reduces stress and anxiety, balances mood, and helps you sleep better. Add 2–3 drops of jasmine essential oil to 15 ml (3 tsp) of a base oil such as grapeseed or jojoba, and massage it into your skin before going to bed.

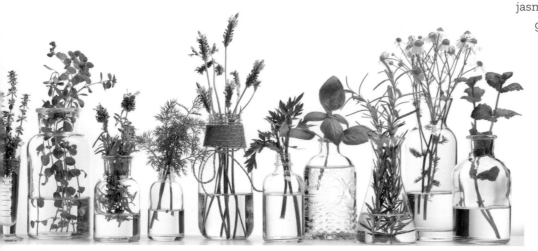

BERGAMOT

"Most people find the sweet, dry citrus aroma of bergamot essential oil very appealing and gently uplifting," says Jo. "It's also good for stress and will leave you feeling more relaxed, so you get a better night's sleep. It combines beautifully with other oils, particularly lavender and chamomile, which are also very calming." Add a few drops of bergamot to an oil diffuser or a pillow spray to evoke a calming, sedative environment before going to bed.

YLANG YLANG

This sweet, exotic, sensual smell is so good they named it twice! "Ylang ylang is best known for its aphrodisiac and mood-enhancing properties," says Christina Salcedas, global director of education at Aromatherapy Associates. "It's also a fantastic sleep tonic. The scent reduces blood pressure and heart rate and eases anxiety, helping you to gently unwind physically and mentally," she says. "For a powerful sleep blend, combine a few drops with sandalwood and clary sage. Or, add two drops of ylang ylang and two drops of vanilla essence or essential oil to 20 ml (3½ tsp) of body butter or lotion, then dab on your wrists, shoulders, and upper chest area," suggests Christina.

CLARY SAGE

The purple flowers of clary sage, grown mainly in the South of France and Italy, emit a rich, musky scent. The essential oil has been shown in studies to calm the nervous system and reduce blood pressure, heart rate, and levels of the stress hormone cortisol. In one study reported in the *Journal of Alternative and Complementary Medicine* in 2012, it was shown that clary sage helped women to feel less anxious before a urological examination. So, it can make a potent aid if your sleep issues are anxiety- or stress-related. You can use clary sage on its own, or blend it with jasmine, lavender, sandalwood, and vetiver.

FRANKINCENSE

This has been used since biblical times as part of holy and ceremonial rituals. Derived from bark resin found in the Middle East, Somalia, Ethiopia, and China, its woody, balsamic scent has a deeply calming, purifying and meditative effect. "The scent of frankincense calms the respiratory system, relaxes the diaphragm, and encourages deeper breathing," says Christina. "It helps to alleviate anxiety and stress. If you have a tendency to wake up in the night, add a drop of frankincense to a tissue, then take a deep breath into it. This will soon help you to get back to sleep."

"You can't look at a sleeping cat and feel tense."
Jane Pauley, television host, journalist and and author

6 WAYS TO WAKE UP REFRESHED

Once you've had your sleep, try these morning fixes to make sure you get out of bed on the right foot every day.

1. Drink a glass of water

Keep some water on your bedside table so you can sip it as soon as you wake up in the morning. This helps to kickstart hydration—good for your mind and body.

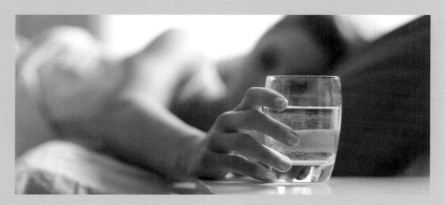

2. Meditate in the morning

"Meditation presses the reset button, allowing you to start each day as a blank canvas," says Steve Chamberlain, life coach and author of *On Purpose*. "It also helps to create separation between you and your thoughts, which can enable you to be more present and focused throughout the day." While it's tempting to meditate from the comfort of your bed, this might not the best idea. "Choose a place that feels comforting or cosy in your house—you could grab a blanket so you're warm. Initially, simply close your eyes, and allow your mind and thoughts to do whatever they want to do, then you can choose to focus on your breath, returning to it each time your mind wanders."

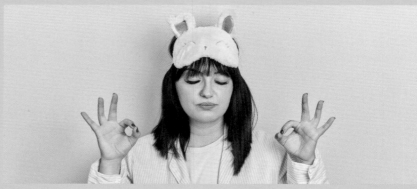

3. Stretch your body

Gently move your body with a short yoga flow or simple stretch—it's a good way of being mindful first thing in the morning. "A morning stretch will start to get your energy flowing and, by consciously focusing your attention on each muscle as you stretch, it allows you to mindfully come into the present moment," says Chamberlain. "Practiced daily, over time you'll notice you have more flexibility and energy throughout your day."

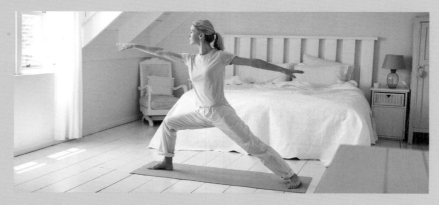

4. Set a positive intention

Your mind is a powerful tool, so program it to help you make the most of the day ahead. "Set an intention for who you choose to be and how you will choose to show up in each moment," suggests Chamberlain. "Life rewards intent and action, so you'll likely start to notice more positive results playing out. Keep your intention short and to the point, which will allow you to easily align with it throughout your day—'I choose to be courageous in everything I do' or 'I am open and present' are good examples of a positive daily intention."

5. Take a cold shower!

Having a cold (or cool) shower, even for just 30 seconds or a minute, has many health benefits, with studies showing it can help with everything from boosting endorphins (the happy hormone), to improving your circulation and supporting your immune system. "It might seem unpleasant, but a cold shower shocks you into the present moment and wakes up all of your senses," says Chamberlain. "Start with a 10-second cold blast before turning to warm and gradually building up."

6. Eat a nutritious breakfast

Often hailed as the most vital meal of the day, eating a nutritious breakfast has been shown to improve concentration, support digestion, and protect your heart. What's more, studies show that your body is better able to process nutrients in the morning, meaning that first meal of the day can have a significant impact on your overall health. Opt for a healthier, more substantial choice, such as porridge topped with fruit, or avocado on seeded toast.

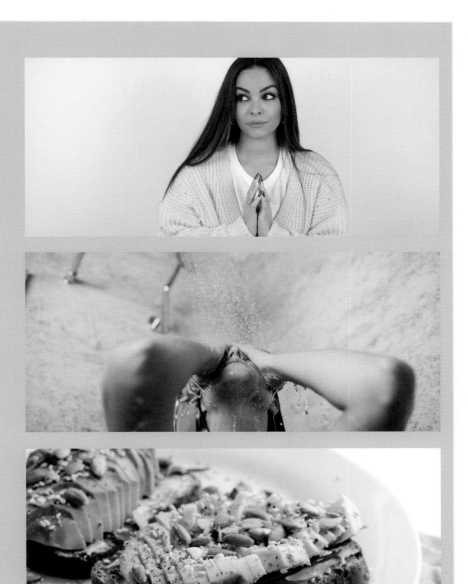

ALTERNATIVE WAYS TO GET MORE ENERGY!

These natural energy boosters will help you feel refreshed and revitalized from the moment you wake up!

When you emerge from a deep sleep, do you still feel like hibernating? "Low energy can occur for many reasons: stress, lack of sleep, poor nutrition, and other lifestyle factors," says Zen master Sandy Taikyu Kuhn Shimu. "But, many people also push themselves too hard. They take on extra work, socialize when they'd rather have a night off, or offer to help out with something because they think they 'have to.' All this can leave you feeling depleted." Luckily there are lots of simple ways to get a natural energy boost. 'You don't have to go on an exotic holiday or be a Zen master—you can feel energized by making small, daily changes,' says Sandy. "Buddhist philosophy teaches that if you practice a healthy ritual for 108 days, it can lead to transformation," she adds. Studies show that even 30 days of repeating the same action can lead to lasting habit changes, so why not make March the month to re-energize your body, mind, and life? Sandy's tips will help you feel invigorated and full of energy and vigor.

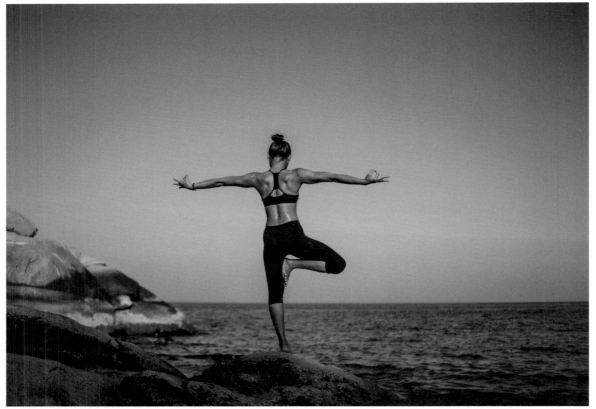

Left: *Eating healthily and doing some deep breathing and regular exercise not only gives you more energy, it also reduces your risk of illness while boosting your self-esteem, mood, and sleep quality.*

DETOX THE AIR
Spritz the air with calming lavender and rosemary essence while also ridding your bedroom of bacteria and dust mites.

REVITALIZE YOUR BREATHING

The way you breathe has a huge impact on your energy. Breathing slowly and deeply maximizes oxygen intake, which increases vitality. Deep, rhythmic breathing also harmonizes and cleanses your whole system, improving concentration and mental clarity.

Try "alternate nostril breathing"

- Breathe in and close your left nostril with your left thumb.
- Breathe out through your right nostril, then inhale through the same nostril.
- Close your right nostril with the little finger and ring finger of your left hand, so that both nostrils are closed.
- Hold your breath for a few seconds, then release your thumb, breathing out through your left nostril.
- Inhale again through your left nostril, then close it with your thumb.
- Hold your breath for a few seconds, release your fingers and breathe out through the right nostril, then in again.
- Repeat eight rounds of this.

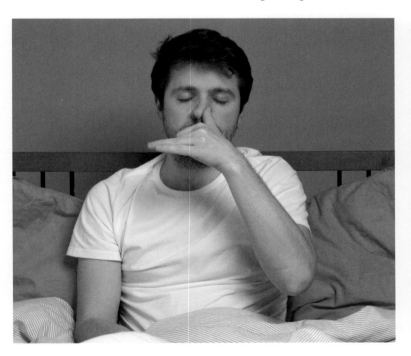 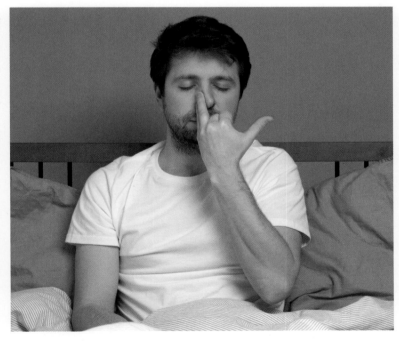

COMPLEMENTARY AND ALTERNATIVE THERAPIES

There are plenty of alternatives to mainstream medicine, many of which have been practiced since ancient times. Note that anyone can carry out these treatments, even without formal qualifications or experience, so do some research to find a practitioner who will carry out your treatment in a way that's acceptable to you. Here are some of the main complementary therapies available:

TRADITIONAL ALTERNATIVE MEDICINE
• Acupuncture, homeopathy, and Oriental practices.

BODY THERAPIES
• Chiropractic and osteopathic medicine, Alexander technique, massage, yoga, Pilates, tai chi, and reflexology.

DIETARY AND HERBAL APPROACHES
• Herbal remedies and supplements, including cannabis-based medicines.

EXTERNAL ENERGY THERAPIES
• Electromagnetic therapy, reiki, and qigong.

MIND THERAPIES
• Meditation, biofeedback, and hypnosis.

SENSE THERAPIES
• Art, dance, music, visualization, and guided imagery.

TAP YOUR THYMUS

Your thymus is located in the upper chest, behind the sternum and about 7 cm (3 in) beneath the throat. It regulates your body's immune system by secreting "defence hormones" (lymphocytes). When your immune system is strong, you have more energy. Tapping the thymus gland is common practice in China, where many people do it first thing in the morning, often in a park before work. Tapping this point also reduces stress and anxiety.

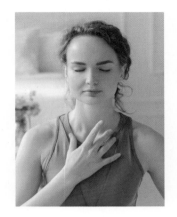

- Stand or sit upright.
- Breathing slowly and deeply, tap on the thymus (sternum) with your fingertips or fist for 60 seconds.
- Do this several times a day for an instant pick-me-up.

MASSAGE YOUR SCALP

Using your fingernails to "comb" your hair stimulates numerous acupuncture points on your scalp. This gets the energy (qi) flowing through your body, clearing stagnation and stimulating the circulation. It has an energizing effect on the mind and body.

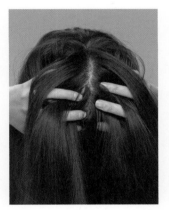

- Using both hands, "comb" your entire scalp with your fingernails.
- Work your way from your hairline over your head and down the back of your neck. Comb in "lines" to make sure you cover your whole head.
- Repeat nine times.

WALK BACKWARDS

This is not something we tend to do in the West, but if you go to China or Japan, you'll find that walking backwards is very popular. There is even an Asian proverb that says: "100 steps backward are worth more than 1,000 steps forward." Walking backwards not only strengthens your energy channels, increasing vitality, but it harmonizes the left and right sides of your brain, improving concentration and balance, stimulating the imagination, and working muscles you don't normally use.

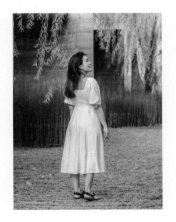

- Before you start, make sure you'll be walking in a safe environment where you won't be bumping into things.
- Start walking backwards in a circle, taking slow, small steps, without looking behind you. Breathe slowly and deeply.
- Do this for a few minutes every day. With practice, you'll feel more confident about walking longer distances in a straight line.

VITALITY SHOT

Skip energy-zapping carbs for breakfast and start your day with this ayurvedic energy drink combining ginger, carrots, beetroot, and lemon, all designed to pep you up.

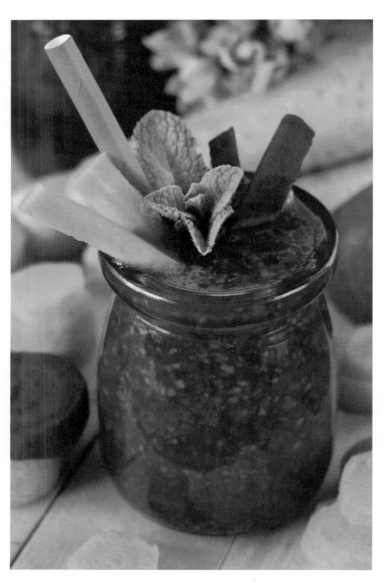

- 3 carrots, chopped
- 1 beetroot, chopped
- ¼ in ginger root
- ½ tbsp lemon juice
- A pinch of ground cardamom
- ½ tbsp maple syrup (optional)

1. Juice the carrots, beetroot, and ginger.
2. Add the lemon juice, cardamom, and maple syrup.
3. Knead or mix into a dough and leave to chill in the fridge for 30 minutes.
4. Process in a blender or just stir, then drink straight away.

FOODS AND DRINKS FOR ENERGY

Here are some of the best sources of energy that will keep you going throughout the day:

Fruits: Bananas, avocados, goji berries, apples, strawberries, oranges, and dark berries.

Vegetables: Yams, sweet potatoes, beetroot, and dark, leafy greens.

Liquids: Water, coffee (in limited amounts), green tea, and yerba maté (a drink native to South America).

SATISFY YOUR SWEET TOOTH

If you're tired, you're more susceptible to snacking on sugary foods. But while a quick sugar hit can have an instant energizing effect, you'll feel more tired as the day goes on. Too much sugar plays havoc with your blood sugar levels, and when these spike then fall, so does your mood and your energy. Next time you crave something sweet, have a "Nerve Cookie" instead.

This recipe is based on Hildegard of Bingen's *Joy Cookies*. Hildegard was a 12th-century medieval mystic and medicine woman. The biscuits contain nutmeg, cinnamon, and cloves—spices that have a restorative effect. Nutmeg contains myristicin and mace lignan, natural organic compounds that have a stimulating effect, supporting focus and concentration. Cinnamon helps to regulate blood sugar, and cloves promote good digestion.

- 400 g (14 oz) spelt flour
- 250 g (8½ oz) butter, cubed
- 100 g (3½ oz) whole cane sugar
- 200 g (7 oz) ground almonds
- 2 eggs, beaten
- 4 tsp ground cinnamon
- 4 tsp grated nutmeg
- 1 tsp ground cloves
- A pinch of salt

1. Place the flour in a bowl.
2. Add the butter, sugar, almonds, eggs, and spices.
3. Knead or mix into a dough and leave to chill in the fridge for 30 minutes.
4. Roll the dough and cut into shapes.
5. Bake for 10–15 minutes in a moderate oven, 180°C/350°F/Gas 4.

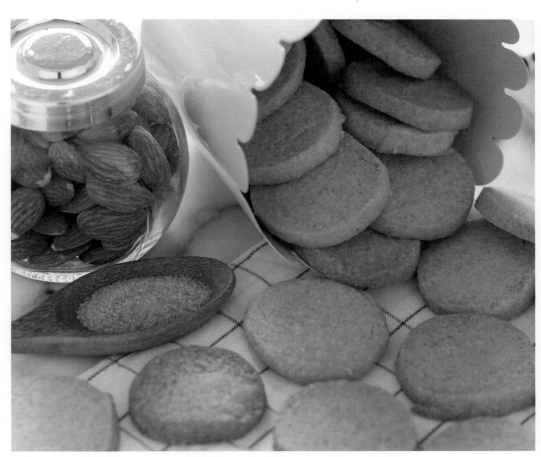

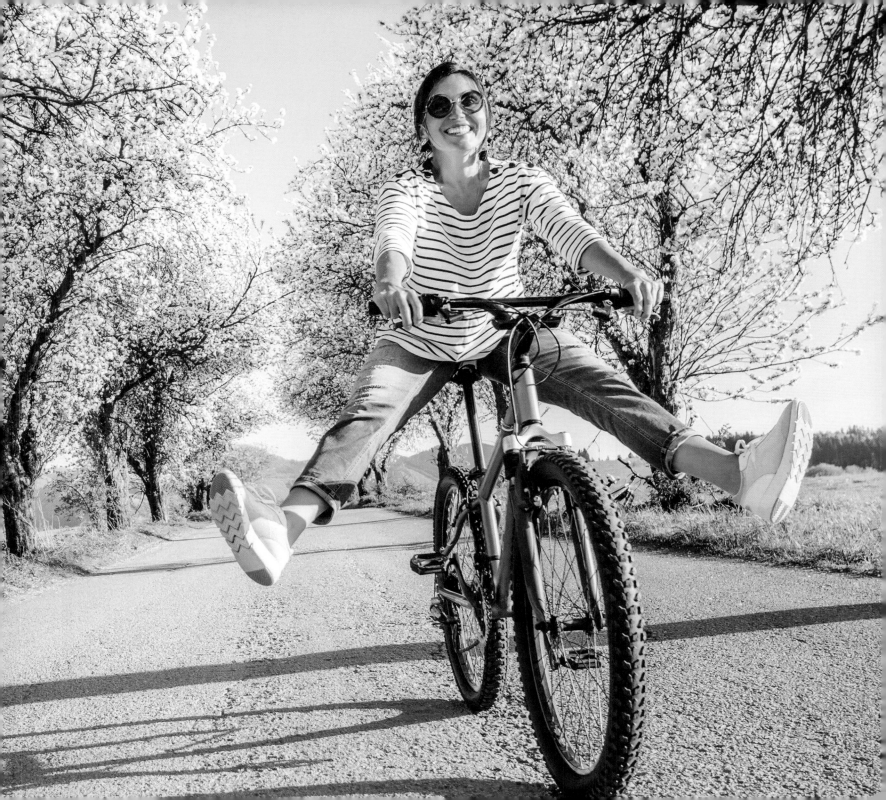

6
HEALTHY AGING

Getting older is a fact of life, but the key to aging well is aging healthily and happily. Having a positive mental attitude is just as important as diet and exercise, so we begin by showing how you can lower your "spirit age" by using positive thinking. There are nutritional and fitness suggestions, some yoga poses to keep you supple, guidance for coping with menopause, and a list of health tips for older men. We close with ways of reducing your risk of dementia, helping you to age as well as possible.

HOW TO AGE WELL

When it comes to staying healthy as you get older, your attitudes and aspirations play as much a part as what you eat and drink. Lynda Gratton and Andrew J. Scott, authors of *The New Long Life*, explain why.

When you think about age, you are usually drawn to your chronological age—the number of candles on your birthday cake. Let's imagine you are 55. Your underlying assumptions are that your chronological age is the go-to measure; that you can look back to your mother at 60 to gain an idea of what the next five years will bring. However, looking at how your mother or grandmother grew older isn't relevant to you. For the past century, every decade has seen people living on average 2–3 years longer than the previous decade. When your grandmother was 55, she probably had fewer than 10 years of healthy living ahead of her. By contrast, you could have more than 30 healthy years to go! Just looking around you, you'll find examples of how people age differently. Perhaps you know of a 70-year-old who runs marathons, and some 50-year-olds who have already slowed down.

The good news is that age is malleable, by which we mean it can be shaped by circumstances and by your own actions, behaviors, and habits. Your DNA actually only accounts for less than a quarter of how you age. This means you can effectively change your age, which is good news! No matter your current age, you have the chance to shape your own future: to learn a new skill, take a new job, build new relationships. Here are a few ways to age well...

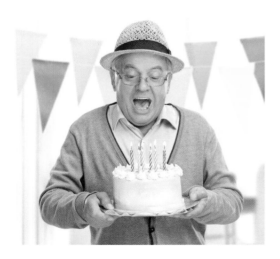 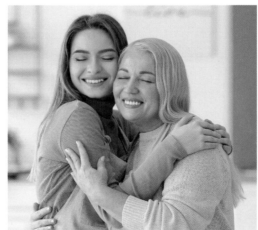 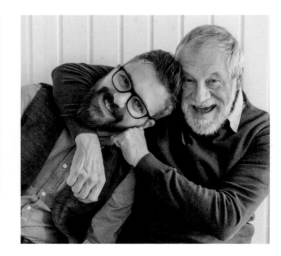

STAY POSITIVE

There is clear evidence that a positive, upbeat mindset has a significant impact on aging well. Emotions really can be contagious, too—it's easy to be deeply affected by the emotions of others—so prioritize spending time with upbeat friends and limit your time with people who complain or just leave you feeling down. Next, spend as much time as possible with people of different ages to you—it's good to be surrounded both by the energy of youth and the wisdom of age. Finally, continue to imagine a positive future. Focus on the person you need to become in order to live that positive future, and where you might need to grow or develop. Think about what would bring you the most pleasure and purpose.

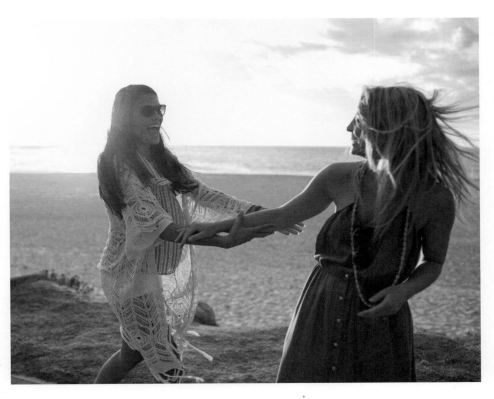

INVEST IN FRIENDSHIPS

An intriguing finding comes from research that looked at a group of people across the whole of their lives—from their student days to old age. One of the questions researchers asked was: "What did those people who led happy lives do?" While one of the answers was that they had enough money—numerous studies show that being poor is a source of unhappiness in old age—what emerged as more crucial was the quality and depth of their friendships. People who were the happiest tended to have invested time in their relationships with family and friends. These bonds become great sources of joy and of solace.

TAKE THE EXERCISE PILL

We started out our research by talking to directors of aging centers across the world. We were interested in how they thought the field of aging research would develop. But we were also intrigued by their own life choices. So, we asked each of them: "What are you doing to age well?" There were some differences in their answers: one used virgin olive oil as often as possible; another fasted one day a week. But what all of them had in common was one simple habit: they all exercised. Some ran, others boxed, some rowed, but they all got their heart rate up a couple of times a week. As one wryly remarked, "If exercise were a pill a company could sell—it would be the richest company in the world."

WHAT IS YOUR "SPIRIT AGE"?

Two of the main determining factors when it comes to how healthy and happy you are in your later years are your mindset and outlook on life. With positive thinking, you can actually slow down the aging process.

When model Christie Brinkley had her 65th birthday, instead of celebrating that actual number, she called it her 15th 50th birthday, in recognition of the fact that she felt no older than 50. This, she said, was her "spirit age," which had nothing to do with how old she might have been chronologically.

Thinking this way has been proven to turn back the clock. In recent years, researchers examining the science of aging have found that the more positive we feel about getting older, the more slowly it happens. People who think they are younger than they are have brains that look and act younger than their peers. And those with positive attitudes to getting older have better health during old age—they even live up to seven-and-a-half years longer than those with less positive beliefs. With arthritis or

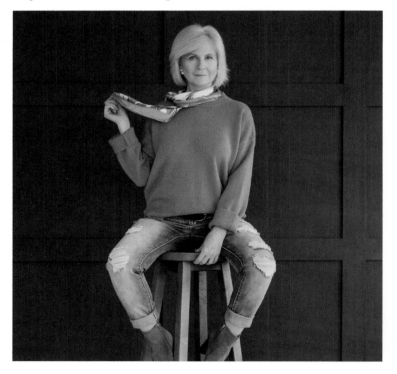

high blood pressure, you shouldn't just think, "Well, that's normal at my age." Instead, you should look for ways to help lessen the condition, such as exercise and changing your diet. "Those with more negative beliefs tend to have a 'what's the point' attitude and just let things take their course," says Dr. Hannah Swift, a researcher on aging psychology at the University of Kent. Negative attitudes to aging are also stressful on your system, which in itself takes its toll. Shockingly, people in a research study who had a negative idea about aging before the age of 39 were twice as likely to have a heart attack after 60—something the researchers attributed to their subjects' stress and anxiety.

> "Your spirit age is how you've kicked around the world. It's what you've gathered and how you move and your point of view, your enthusiasm, your gratitude, your appreciation. It's your energy, your aura—that's your true age. Not that other arbitrary number."
> Christie Brinkley, model and actress

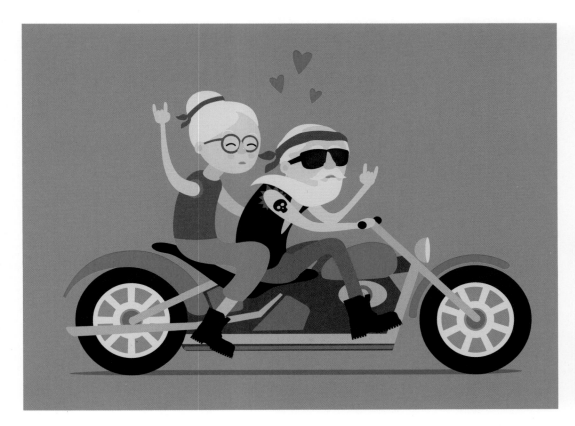

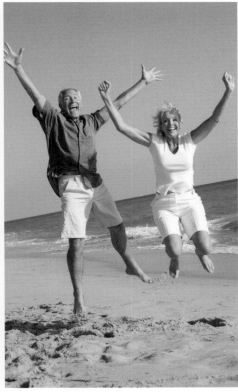

YOUR TIME IS NOW!

Our attitudes to aging are set in childhood, "but our 40s and 50s are a real flashpoint for them coming to the surface," says psychotherapist and self-esteem coach Alison Moore (bemoore.uk). "One reason for this is the approach of menopause—so many women link youth to fertility that as menopause approaches, it makes us think more about our age. We start to worry about what others think; we start to wonder whether we're too old to wear this or do that and we start to feel we need to conform."

   Here's where having a "spirit age" comes in handy, as it helps to counteract all of this... but, how do you find it? For some, it's easy—it's that number that flashes unbidden into your head when someone asks how old you are. For others, you might need to ask yourself a few questions about how much younger or older you feel than your peers? What age do you feel inside? What age do others think you are? All of these things combined create the attitude and feeling that make up your spirit age. So read on to find out how to stay young at heart.

6 WAYS TO LOWER YOUR SPIRIT AGE

The following practical tips from Dr. Hannah Swift and Alison Moore will help you to lower your spirit age and help you feel more vital, invigorated and rejuvenated in both mind and body.

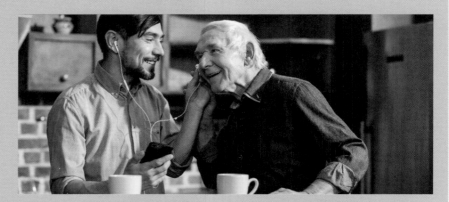

1. Spend time with youthful thinkers

If all your friends are starting to wear ankle-length trousers and flat shoes and moan about "the youth of today," you can be inclined to think the same way. "It's natural for you to want to fit in with your friends, so look at who you mostly mix with and make sure they inspire your new positive attitude," says Alison.

2. But also know where you're comfortable

Sometimes, being around younger folk may do more harm than good. It's known as "stereotype threat," which Hannah explains as a situation where your confidence gets sapped because you feel out of place. This can unconsciously cause you to perform worse than you should. "In studies on brain health, people told they were going to be compared with younger people performed worse than normal," says Hannah. If you feel like this in an area of your life, improving your self-belief in the area will help, but while you work on that, stay in your comfort zone.

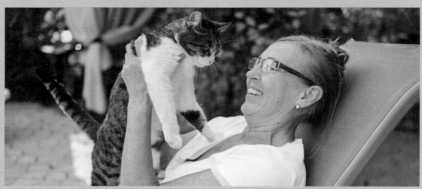

3. Try new experiences

According to studies, seniors who stay young at heart are more open to doing new things. Don't fall into ruts such as eating the same foods or visiting the same places all the time. Being inquiring and curious keeps your brain working and keeps you young.

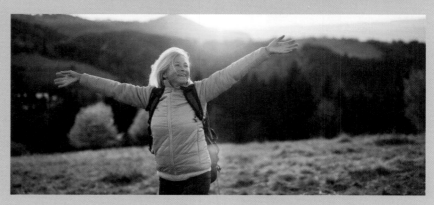

4. Check your perceptions

Unfortunately, some people subconsciously equate aging to infirmity and weakness, making the assumption that getting older automatically heralds the onset of conditions such as deafness, immobility, and long-term illness. "One of the reasons we fear getting older is because of the way we perceive the elderly in general—as a bit hopeless and helpless. But ask yourself whether this is your reality," says Alison. "Chances are it's not, so don't reinforce it." Never listen to people who say things like, "She ought to act her age." If you want to dye your hair pink, go out dancing in clubs, and travel the world, do it!

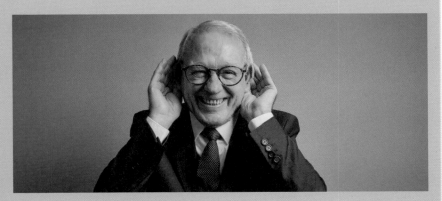

5. Pick the right role models

Finding role models that challenge your beliefs about aging also helps you settle in to your spirit age. But you need the right role models. Surprisingly, Googling "90-year-olds running marathons" might not actually help. "This type of behavior is usually presented as extraordinary, which may actually reinforce negative stereotypes," says Hannah. Instead, just look for people challenging negative images of aging in less extreme ways. Think of the men and women still playing tennis at their local court in their 70s, rather than 90-year-olds running marathons.

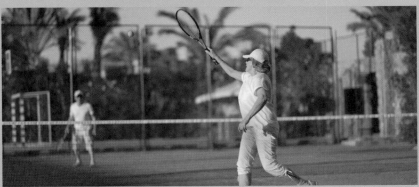

6. Celebrate your birthdays!

If you stop marking your birthdays, you're telling your mind that this is something you're ashamed of. "Embrace the fact you had another great year!" says Alison. Why not start planning your next party now?

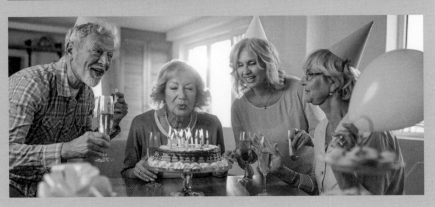

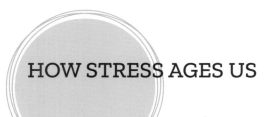

HOW STRESS AGES US

We've discussed stress in an earlier chapter, but it's worth returning to here as a reminder of its harmful effects as we age. Stress will make you look and feel older—and the only way to prevent this from happening is to reduce or eliminate its source. When you read this, you'll want to do just that...

We all know that too much stress is bad for us, but you may not know that it also ages us from the inside. Thousands of years ago, our ancestors faced serious threats to their lives on a regular basis. To them, stress meant being in imminent danger, usually the risk of being eaten by an animal or having to fight others. Nowadays, most of the threats we face are more likely to be emotional or mental stressors. When we face stressful situations, our bodies produce adrenaline in response to a perceived threat and the following process occurs:

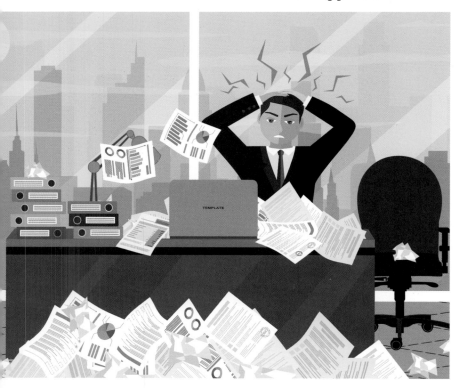

- Blood is diverted to the brain, heart, lungs, and muscles, which need to work harder to get you out of danger.
- The heart rate speeds up to pump blood more effectively around the body to these areas.
- Blood is diverted away from the digestive tract, as stopping to eat isn't on the agenda when it's a matter of life or death.
- Breathing speeds up to get oxygen to the muscles as quickly as possible.
- Sweat levels go up to stop the body from overheating.
- Blood sugar levels increase dramatically so that glucose is available to feed the brain and muscles.
- Blood vessels constrict, so blood pressure goes up.
- Your senses become more acute to enable you to pick up as much information as possible in order to make good judgements.

The body also produces cortisol, a steroid hormone produced in response to stress. This will make the stress response last longer, causing long-term health issues. Alison Cullen, nutritional therapist from A. Vogel says: "If this goes on for long periods of time, this impacts our long-term health. Growth and reproduction (in the body) are halted. Immune function is focused on countering wounds, so patrolling to spot infections and tumors and so on is put on hold. Your risk of getting infections goes up and you are less able to defend yourself against any disease processes already artwork in your body."

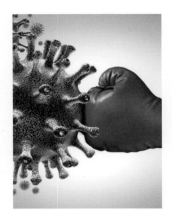

Alison adds: "No surplus energy is stored, so fatigue is more likely. Bone formation and mending is neglected, blood pressure rises and damages blood vessels, blood becomes more viscous (and is more likely to form clots), and food metabolism is affected."

Stress can also affect your ability to digest food. "Blood flow is directed away from digestion and from the skin—you become pale and tired-looking and can't easily absorb nutrients from your food," says Alison. "When the stress is purely psychological, the stress response can become more damaging than the stressor itself because the chemicals produced to enable us to run or fight aren't burnt off."

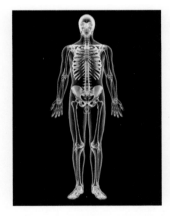

During prolonged periods of stress, your body also ages faster. "Long-term exposure to cortisol causes delayed wound healing, muscle weakness, increased risk of infection, inhibition of bone formation, and suppression of calcium absorption," warns Alison. "We are lower in the nutrients we need, and oxygen is not circulating efficiently to our skin, so wastes are not being efficiently removed from the skin." Chronic stress can undermine your immune system, interfere with your sleep, and therefore stop your body from repairing itself properly. It also affects weight and digestion.

DON'T IGNORE STRESS!

If you've coped with a very stressful situation, don't forget you may pay a price for it later on, even when the stress has supposedly gone. "Many women cope extraordinarily well during times of crisis, and don't suffer the consequences for a long time afterwards," says Alison. "Post-traumatic stress is now recognized, but many people assume it only affects people who have faced trauma. Actually, long-drawn out stresses, such as caring for a terminally ill parent/partner/child, can be just as impactful on the nervous system and involve a long recovery time. The nervous system has become so used to being on [edge] that it takes a lot of peaceful time to convince it to come down off red alert."

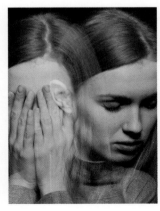

30 WAYS TO LOOK YOUNG AND STAY HEALTHY

There's a lot you can do to look and feel healthy. Adjusting your diet, exercising regularly, and making the right lifestyle choices all make a big difference. Here's a summary of dos and don'ts.

REDUCE YOUR EXPOSURE TO THE SUN

Don't spend too long in the sun—its ultraviolet light damages elastin (the fibers in the skin), leading to facial wrinkles. Too much sun can also cause freckles, destruction of elastic and collagen tissue (causing more lines and wrinkles), and, more worryingly, skin cancer.

WEAR SUNSCREEN ALL YEAR ROUND

It doesn't matter whether it's winter or summer, wearing a sunscreen of at least SPF 30 will help to combat the signs of aging by reducing the effect of ultraviolet rays on the skin.

EXFOLIATE DAILY

Using a simple face scrub regularly can give you a clearer and more youthful complexion. Don't forget your hands, too, as these are often a giveaway when it comes to age!

GET ENOUGH SLEEP

Work out how much you need personally for optimum health (most of us need 6–8 hours a night). Go to bed 30 minutes or an hour earlier each night if you can. Keep technology out of the bedroom, too, so that you're more likely to get to sleep more easily.

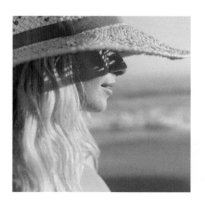
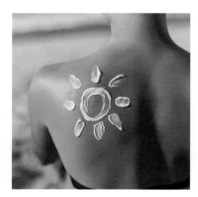
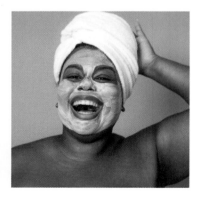
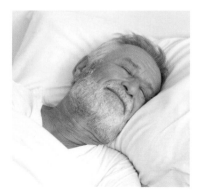

DON'T BE TOO THIN

Our cheeks start to lose their plumpness when we reach our late 30s. If you're on a strict diet, you're likely to lose a lot of weight from your face, which makes your cheeks hollow and gives an older appearance. Losing and gaining weight in a yo-yo dieting fashion will also age you, as ligaments in the face can be stretched and then become looser, resulting in more nose-to-mouth lines.

GET THE RIGHT HAIRSTYLE

Hairstyles where the hair appears thin and fine—for example when hair is long and straight with no texture or layers—can make women look aged and unhealthy. "Long, flat hair can also make the face look drawn and any sagging areas more noticeable," says Sarah McKenna, owner of Vixen & Blush hair salons in London.

LOOK AFTER YOUR TEETH

The state of your teeth affects your overall health, as gum disease can increase your risk of stroke, diabetes, and heart disease (gum disease can cause inflammation that can lead to damaged blood vessels in the heart). Be sure to visit the dentist regularly, brush your teeth at least twice a day and floss daily.

GET A PET

In a study published on www.petplace.com, a researcher at the State University of New York at Buffalo found that stockbrokers with high blood pressure who adopted a cat or a dog had lower blood pressure readings when they encountered stress compared to those who didn't have a pet.

AVOID POLLUTION AND SMOKE

- Don't exercise in busy, polluted environments, or spend too long in these areas. Oxidative damage occurs when we spend too much time exposed to polluted air.
- Don't smoke. Smoking is a leading cause of premature wrinkles, as it affects the blood supply that keeps the skin looking supple. It can also stain your teeth and make them look yellow. Avoid being in areas where other people are smoking, too.
- Avoid processed, barbecued, smoked, or overcooked foods. All of these contain cancer-causing chemicals, and not eating them can help to reduce your intake of free radicals.

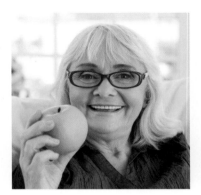
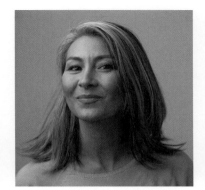
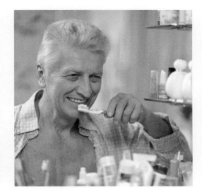
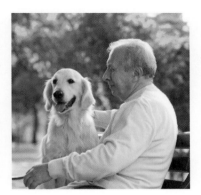

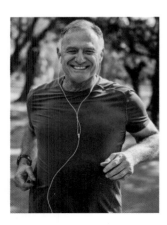

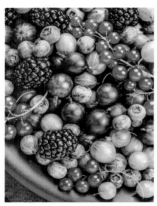

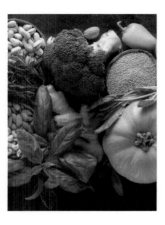

HAVE A REGULAR EXERCISE ROUTINE

Consistency pays off, so organize a weekly exercise routine that works for you. Researchers at McMaster University in Ontario found that even people who started to exercise later in life had younger skin than those who didn't exercise.

DON'T OVEREAT

While we don't recommend very strict diets, eating too many calories can cause aging and push blood sugar levels up too high. Restricting calories is thought to slow down the aging process, as it seems to lower levels of glucose, insulin, and cholesterol levels, but don't restrict your intake by more than 40 percent. Cutting calories by 25 percent of the recommended daily intake (2,500 for men; 2,000 for women) is more sensible, or consuming just under the recommended guidelines could be helpful.

TAKE MORE ANTIOXIDANTS

Make sure your diet includes plenty of antioxidants, which neutralize free radicals that can cause sun damage and wrinkles. Try blueberries, strawberries, artichokes, goji berries, kale, and pecans.

TAKE A VITAMIN D SUPPLEMENT

This calcium-regulating hormone helps to regulate the amount of calcium and phosphate in the body, keeping our bones, teeth, and muscles healthy. It also helps us to maintain healthy brain function, avoid age-related eye disease, and provides protection from cancer, heart disease, and infections.

DRINK EIGHT GLASSES OF WATER EVERY DAY

Water flushes waste out of your system and helps transport nutrients around the body. It also regulates metabolism, which can prevent weight gain. Drinking plenty of water can help to keep your skin looking good, too, as dehydration can make it look dry and wrinkled.

GO GREEN

Green tea is rich in antioxidants, so try to drink a cup every day. Antioxidants help to protect skin from free radical damage. In a study of women, those who drank at least five cups of green tea daily had a 42 percent lower risk of death due to stroke than those who drank less than one cup per day.

GET ENOUGH MAGNESIUM

This important mineral helps to boost mood, memory, and thinking power, as it is involved in nerve signaling at junctions between cells. Good sources include kelp, seaweed, squash, pumpkin seeds, steamed broccoli, and halibut.

EAT MORE...

Fish: Consume more oily fish such as salmon, tuna, mackerel, or herring. Oily fish contains essential fatty acids that help to protect skin cell membranes and stop the skin from getting too dry. Oily fish also protects your joints and boosts your brain function.

Brightly colored vegetables: Aim to include a wide range of bright colors on your plate, such as red, orange, and yellow (bell) peppers.

Tomatoes: These contain an antioxidant called lycopene, which gives them their red color and helps to breakdown free radicals—by-products produced by the body that can stress our bodies and cause aging and cell damage.

Protein: Two key proteins in the skin—collagen and elastin—make up the dermis, which provides support and structure for your skin. Get your protein from meat, eggs, dairy, and nuts.

Anti-inflammatory foods: Good sources are turmeric and cayenne pepper. These not only help to ease inflammation, they also add tasty flavor to meals.

DITCH...

Sugar: If you eat too much sugar, the sugar in your bloodstream attaches to proteins to form harmful new molecules called Advanced Glycation End Products (AGEs). As they build up, they damage other proteins in a domino-style fashion. This goes on to damage collagen and elastin, which are the protein fibers that keep your skin firm and toned. Once they are damaged, they became dry, and this leads to wrinkles.

Processed foods: These tend to be high in sugar, which contains no nutrients and can increase weight gain. They are often high in refined carbohydrates, too, which can lead to rapid spikes in blood sugar levels. This means that cravings can strike and lead to overeating, causing further weight gain. Many processed foods are also low in nutrients, whereas real foods contain vitamins and minerals.

Alcohol: This dehydrates the body (and therefore the skin) and also interferes with sleep quality, which can prevent your body from repairing and recovering fully. Alcohol can also lead to inflammation in the body, which results in aging.

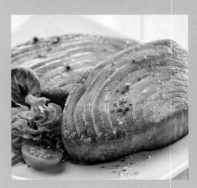 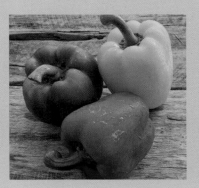 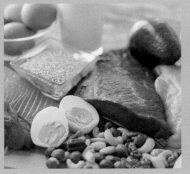 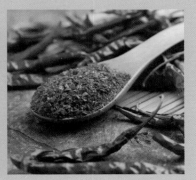

EXERCISE SOLUTIONS FOR CHANGING BODIES

Changes occur in our body as we age, and some of these changes start occurring from the age of 30. The good news is that regular exercise can offset many of them, along with a healthy diet. Here are some of the main physical changes that take place as we get older, with exercise solutions that will help.

MUSCLE MASS

From about the age of 30, our bodies lose lean tissue and muscles begin to shrink. There is a loss of muscle tissue in all areas that is progressive. According to YMCA Fit, an average loss of 30 percent of muscle mass is experienced between the ages of 30 and 80. This is 5 percent per decade. Strength and power are also affected. Reduced muscle mass often means your metabolic rate will slow down because muscle is metabolically active (in other words, it burns calories even at rest.)

Solution: Regular strength training, such as lifting weights or doing a Body Pump class.

BONE DENSITY

Like any other living tissue, our bones constantly change. Calcium is deposited and reabsorbed in a cyclical process from birth to death. Calcium and mineral salts are deposited to maintain strength, and old bone formation is removed to avoid brittle bones. From about the age of 35, peak bone mass and bone density decline about 1 percent each year, affecting women in particular. Bones become more brittle and are more prone to breaking. By around age 70, the female skeleton will have lost around 30 percent of its calcium. After the menopause, bone mass losses of 3–5 percent per year can occur.

Solution: Regular weight-bearing exercise, such as running or strength training.

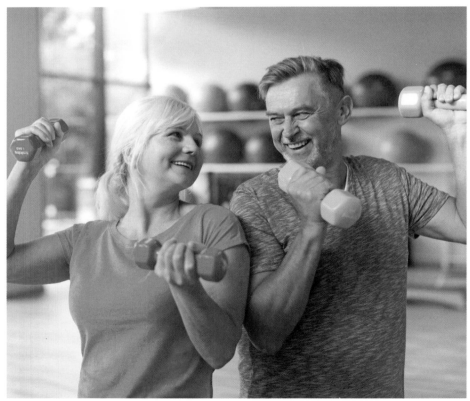

BODY FAT LEVELS

Some people find that their metabolic rate slows down from the age of 30–40 onward, and body fat shifts from around the skin to more evenly over the body and around the internal organs. This is called visceral fat, and it is this type of fat that can increase the risk of heart disease and stroke.

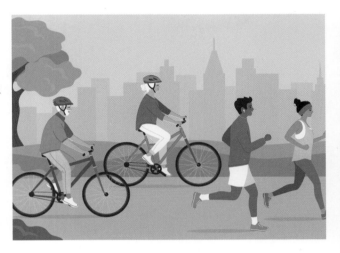

Solution: Regular cardio exercise to burn calories such as running, swimming, cycling, or any other form of exercise that raises your heart rate and makes you moderately out of breath, as well as maintaining a healthy diet.

SKELETAL CHANGES

The skeleton can suffer an increased risk of spinal curvatures, which leads to an increased risk of falls and bad posture. Degenerative changes affect the discs and vertebrae. We lose height and become dehydrated.

Solution: Regular exercise can increase bone mineral density and slow down the aging of the skeleton.

ESTROGEN LEVELS DURING THE MENOPAUSE

In women, the ovaries gradually stop making the hormone estrogen during menopause, which means that production of cortisol and insulin increases. Both of these changes can lead to weight gain, especially around the middle of the body.

Solution: Stay active, keep burning calories, and improve your diet.

ELASTICITY IN CONNECTIVE TISSUE

As we age, the loss of calcium and water leads to a reduction of elasticity in our connective tissue. This causes ligaments and tendons to become brittle and stiff, leading to a reduced range of movement.

Solution: Take up yoga or Pilates to improve flexibility and reduce stiffness.

HOW TO CONTROL AGE-RELATED WEIGHT GAIN

Muscle is metabolically active, enabling our bodies to burn more calories at rest, so the reason why many of us tend to gain weight when we get older is because we lose our muscle mass. Here's what to do about it:

- Be honest about your activity levels. Do you exercise less and spend more time sitting on the sofa? Keep a note of how much you exercise each week. Make sure you meet the recommended activity levels of three to five times per week for 20–90 minutes each time.
- Strength train twice a week to build lean muscle tissue and therefore keep your body more metabolically active.
- To keep your metabolic rate elevated, add high-intensity interval training (HIIT) to your workout schedule once or twice per week if you're already exercising (but not if you're a beginner.)
- Pick four cardio exercises (such as squats, lunges, jumping jacks, and push-ups) and do each one for 20 seconds, having ten seconds' rest in between each exercise, then repeat the circuit eight more times.
- Fill up on healthy foods and increase your protein intake to prevent cravings.

OUTRUN YOUR AGE

Running is a fabulous form of exercise at any age—it's good for both your physical and mental health, improving your cardiovascular system and helping you cope with stress. It's a great all-round way to stay strong as you get older.

THE EXERCISE EFFECT

In recent years, science has shown that many of the physical effects we once thought were caused by aging—weaker muscles, wider waists, easy-to-damage bones—are partially the result of inactivity. Indeed, sporty people have thicker bones than those who sweat less, and they also have longer telomeres (the protective caps at the ends of chromosomes, which protect DNA from deterioration and

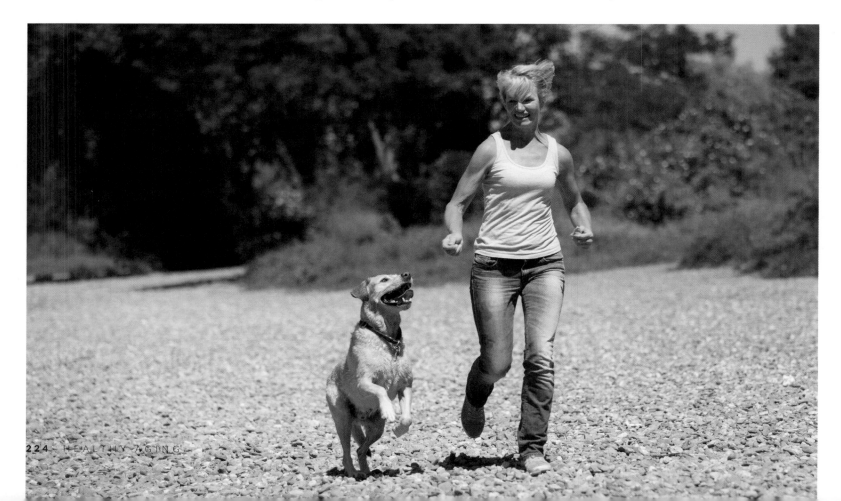

get shorter as you age). "You can lose up to 10 percent muscle mass every decade after 50, but exercise can counteract it," says Dr. Rebecca Robinson, consultant physician in sport and exercise medicine at The Centre for Health and Human Performance (chhp.com). "Older people can get the same response to exercise that a much younger person might have."

WHY RUNNING MATTERS

Clearly, exercise helps in the quest for a youthful body, but does the type of activity you do matter? A bank of science suggests it does. In fact, the latest research published in the *European Heart Journal* reveals that running offers big benefits when it comes to building an ageless body. The German scientists compared different types of workouts—endurance training (distance running), HIIT training (interval running) and resistance training (circuit exercise on gym machines)—and found that running slowed or reversed cellular aging, even when weight training did not. "Metabolically, running is really good for you," adds Dr. Robinson. "It's important to maintain heart- and lung-

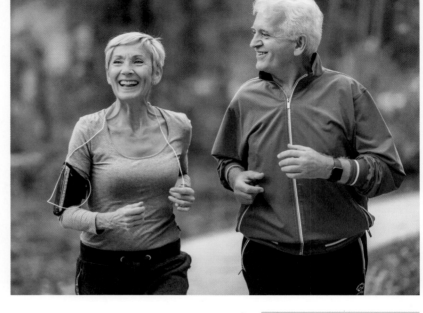

based fitness as you age, and running is great for the cardiovascular system." Further science shows that satellite cells, which help repair and regenerate muscle tissue, are hardier among runners. Plus, runners' muscles are more densely packed with motor units (the muscles' control mechanisms, which can reduce in number as we age) than sedentary types.

GIVE ME STRENGTH

It's important not to discount other forms of activity, especially for women. "After women go through the menopause, they lose the protective effect that hormones have on bone strength, and running can help boost bone density," adds Dr. Robinson. "However, bones like to be loaded in different directions, so supplementing some runs with resistance exercise or Pilates is a really good idea."

If you've been avoiding pounding the pavement because you believe it can cause saggy jowls, droopy breasts, or painful knees and ankles, let's put those rumors to rest. "Running gets a bad reputation for causing things such as joint pain, when it's simply a matter of being holistically strong by complementing runs with strength work," explains Dr. Robinson. And as for saggy skin? "There are some things we need to be mindful of, such as ensuring our bra fits, because running can cause some stretching of the ligaments around the breast, but the rest simply isn't true."

"As every runner knows, running is about more than just putting one foot in front of the other; it is about our lifestyle and who we are."
Joan Benoit Samuelson, first women's Olympic Games marathon champion

GARDENING

As well as taking part in vigorous forms of exercise, such as running, cycling, and swimming, the more relaxing pursuit of gardening is also a highly beneficial activity as we get older. Here are some of the benefits:

• **Strengthens our bones, muscles, and joints:** The physical activity that goes with gardening gives a complete body workout and increases flexibility and strength. It also improves balance, resulting in fewer falls.

• **Reduces the risk of heart disease and stroke:** Spending an enjoyable few hours working in a garden lowers our stress levels and promotes relaxation, keeping our blood pressure at bay and our heart healthy.

• **Connects us with nature and makes us feel happy:** The scents, sights and sounds of flowers, trees, insects, birds, and animals provide stimulation and connection with nature, giving us feelings of peace, positivity, and wellbeing.

• **Improves our environment:** As well as making our own patch more beautiful and providing home-grown produce to enjoy, gardening is good for the planet. Plants give out oxygen and help to reduce pollution, and a diverse ecosystem benefits essential pollinators such as bees, wasps, moths, butterflies, and beetles.

A love of gardening can continue well into old age, even in the face of mobility challenges and other issues. There are plenty of gardening tools and methods specially designed for older people—gardens can be made more accessible by installing raised beds, pathways, and seating, for example, or by using containers. Most nurseries are happy to give advice about which plants are easiest to grow without too much maintenance, so a love of gardening can carry on for a whole lifetime.

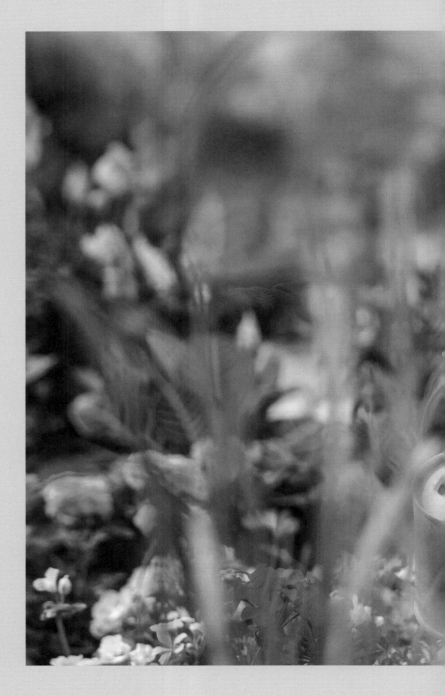

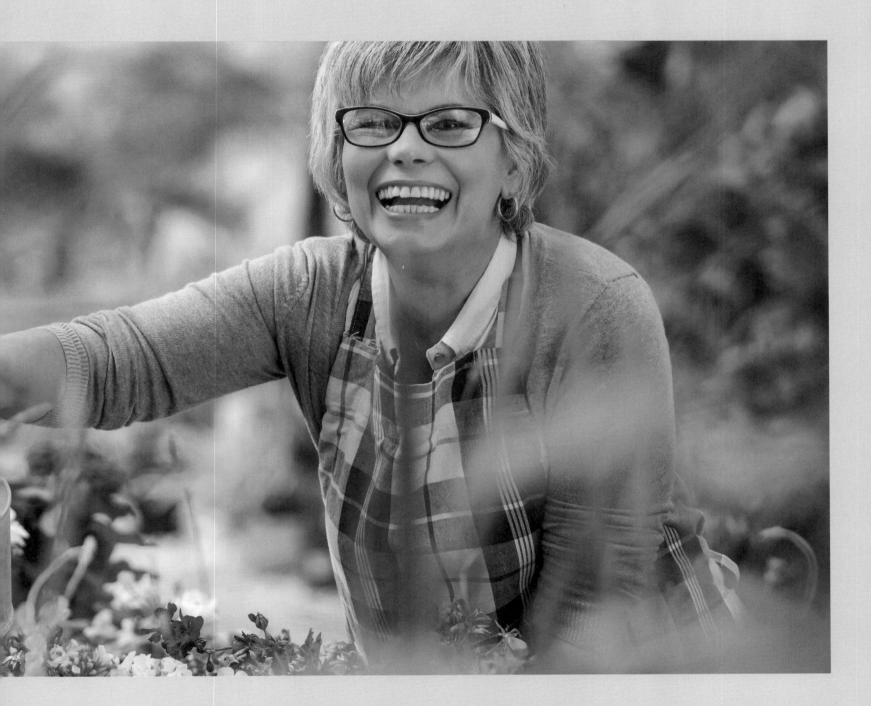

POWER UP YOUR CELLS!

Exercising, receiving a massage, enjoying a coffee or a wine or two, and tweaking meal timings could be the key to feeling younger for longer, as they all help power up your body on a super-cellular level.

What if the key to staying healthy and feeling young were down to something so tiny that a single cell could contain thousands of them? Well, this could be the case—we're talking about your mitochondria, and scientists believe their health is one of the major triggers controlling how you age. In 2016, researchers at Newcastle University removed the mitochondria from aging cells, and this had the effect of turning back time—the cells repaired more quickly than before and produced lower levels of inflammatory chemicals and free radicals. In fact, the scientists said the cells acted like young cells. The reduction in inflammation and free radicals alone is good news for aging, as it reduces the damage that makes you feel older and sicker faster. But surprisingly, it isn't thought to be the main reason why looking after your mitochondria might positively affect how you age; the main benefit is related to the role that mitochondria play in creating energy to power your cells.

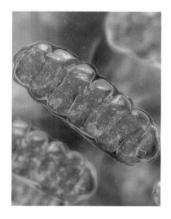

MITOCHONDRIAL HEALTH

Every cell in your body relies on your energy and, therefore, so do all the organs and tissues made up from those cells, such as your skin, heart, and muscles. When mitochondria are producing energy effectively, your body functions optimally—if they're not, things slow down. It's this slow-down that's the cause of most forms of aging. So, keeping your mitochondria firing on all cylinders could potentially help you bypass some of the diseases or other elements of poor health we often associate with old age. "Mitochondrial dysfunction is associated with many of these," says Amanda Sathyapala, clinical senior lecturer at the National Heart and Lung Institute at Imperial College London. "For example, poor functioning in the mitochondria is associated with cells in the liver or fat stores not responding effectively to insulin, which is linked to obesity and type 2 diabetes. Mitochondrial dysfunction in muscle cells results in muscles fatiguing prematurely during exercise and also impairs muscle growth, which can lead to frailty and falls as you get older. When the heart muscle is involved, it's also associated with heart disease."

Looking after the mitochondria may lower your cancer risk, too, as they produce energy for your cells to repair themselves from damage from ultraviolet (UV) rays, pollutants in the air, or cigarette smoke and alcohol. "When a cell is beyond repair, the mitochondria trigger it to die," says Dr. Sathyapala. But by keeping mitochondria healthy, you could reduce the risk of this occurring.

5 WAYS TO POWER UP YOUR CELLS

1. Try high-intensity interval training (HIIT)

Exercise is powered by energy in your muscle cells. When your body notices energy levels becoming depleted, it responds by making more mitochondria. "All types of exercise cause this to happen, but high-intensity interval training generates mitochondria in less time than slower, longer bouts of aerobic exercise," says Dr. Sathyapala. While this might sound as though you need to "go hard or go home" at every workout, recent studies have suggested that for optimum health you need at least two days' recovery between HIIT sessions. "Personally, I suggest people do a variety of different types of exercise—steady state cardio, resistance training and HIIT—throughout the week for promoting mitochondrial number and health," says Dr. Sathyapala.

2. Book a post-workout massage

A 10-minute massage after exercise further increases the growth of new mitochondria, according to a study from the Buck Institute for Research on Aging in California. Researchers believe that the massage reduces levels of inflammatory compounds in your body, thereby lessening any inflammation that could interfere with the way mitochondria behave.

3. Eat and drink resveratrol

The antioxidant resveratrol is found in red grapes and wine, blueberries, and peanuts, and has been found in some early studies to increase mitochondrial numbers. So, why not add a serving or two of foods rich in resveratrol to your diet each day?

4. Keep having your morning coffee

It's been discovered that caffeine causes an enzyme called P27 to move into the mitochondria. It plays an important role in cell repair and was found in a recent German study to protect heart cells from damage and to spark activity in fibroblasts—cells that make structural tissues, including skin and heart muscle.

5. Try intermittent fasting

Dr. Santhypala suggests reducing calorie intake by around 25 percent over the course of the day or trying intermittent fasting where you leave a gap of 12–16 hours between meals. Both have been shown to positively affect mitochondria by reducing the number of free radicals they are exposed to and, in the case of fasting, actually triggering them to stay in a "youthful" state for longer. If calorie restriction doesn't sound appealing, try to at least limit sugar. High levels of sugar in your blood negatively affect mitochondria.

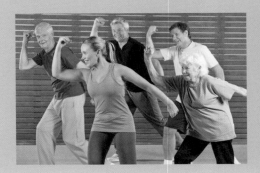
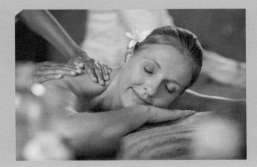
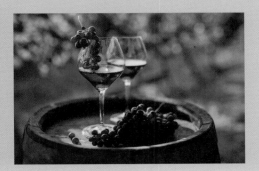

WHY TRY YOGA?

The anti-aging benefits of yoga are clear—you'll be more flexible, have better posture and gain greater strength around your joints—and you're never too old to reap the rewards. Here's some advice on how to get started.

There are so many reasons to try yoga. Not only is it beneficial for improving flexibility and posture—which will help you look younger and slimmer—but also for relaxing the mind and body. Yoga will also help reduce your stress levels. Stress raises your heart rate, increasing the speed at which you age. Yoga helps to calm the mind and makes it easier to manage stress and alleviate depression. Yoga teacher Sheila Maubec (www.shaktishalayogaguernsey.com) says: "Yoga improves strength, stamina, flexibility, joint freedom, range of motion, concentration, and cardiovascular health, and it reduces stress and tension, and tightness in the body and mind. Yoga is about learning to pay attention, direct energy, concentrate on the present moment, and shut out distraction so that every movement becomes meditation."

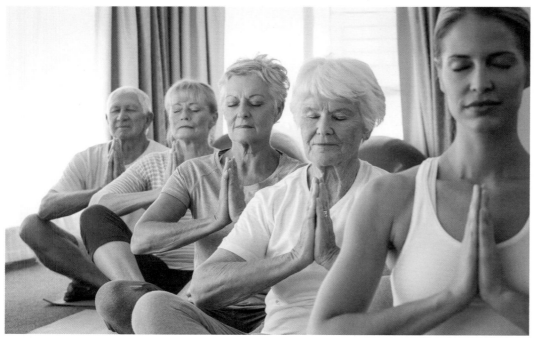

There is good evidence that joint health can be improved greatly through yoga. A 2011 study published in the *Archives Of Gerontology and Geriatrics* showed that those who practiced yoga had much better range of motion while performing everyday tasks compared to those who didn't do yoga.

Yoga is also said to help prevent and relieve the symptoms of arthritis. Staying at a stable body weight and having good flexibility are both thought to help reduce the risk of arthritis, so you can see why yoga would be beneficial.

Practicing yoga can also help to reduce your risk of back problems, as it strengthens your core, which protects your back. Some 80 percent of people experience back pain at some point in their lives, so it's worth doing all you can to look after your back.

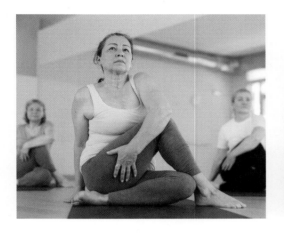
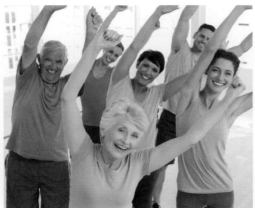
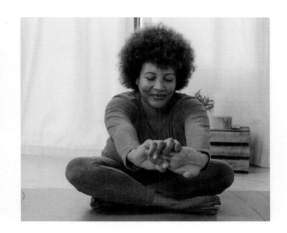

HOW TO GET STARTED

Going to a yoga class will build your confidence. A good instructor will check your technique and adjust your body when necessary, so that you get the most benefit from each pose. Good beginners' classes include **Hatha yoga**, which focuses more on breathing and is a gentle, slower class, and **Iyengar yoga**, which is also slow paced and uses blocks and belts to help you get into the poses correctly. You might also want to try **Kripalu yoga**, which offers gentle and slow movements.

If you want to use yoga to help with weight loss, the faster-paced classes for those who are reasonably fit include:

- **Ashtanga yoga:** A popular favurite with many celebrities who use it to stay in shape.
- **Bikram yoga:** Also called hot yoga—which has 26 poses performed twice, and two breathing exercises.
- **Power yoga:** A challenging and athletic form of yoga based on the poses found in Ashtanga yoga. It builds upper body strength, as well as flexibility and balance.
- **Vinyasa yoga:** Consists of dance-like movements. It focuses on the alignment of the body and building both strength and stamina.

Sheila Maubec says: "Vinyasa, Ashtanga and other forms of Power yoga are the best for weight loss because they are more energetic and work specifically on strength and stamina as well as flexibility. All yoga speeds up the metabolism by stimulating the endocrine glands that regulate metabolic rate. Some more than others. Vinyasa is made up of a series of sun salutations that you move through quickly, so in theory you will increase heart rate, burn calories, and lose weight. The faster pace will increase your resting metabolic rate, which means you will burn more calories."

FIND A GOOD TEACHER
If you do decide to go to a yoga class, ensure you find a good teacher whom you feel comfortable with. It doesn't matter what your level of ability is, a good yoga teacher should be able to put you at ease straight away. They should ask if you have any injuries and also be able to adjust you to improve your alignment without pushing you beyond your capabilities.

YOGA POSES TO KEEP YOU SUPPLE

These yoga poses will strengthen your body and improve your flexibility.

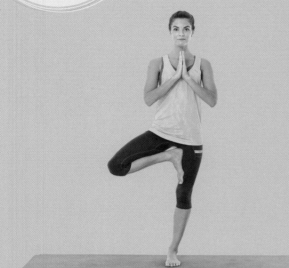

TREE POSE (*left*)
AREAS TRAINED: INNER AND OUTER THIGHS, HIPS, BOTTOM, CORE

Technique

Stand on one leg, press your hands firmly together in front of your chest, and release the tension in your shoulders. Draw the other leg up and place the sole of your foot against the inner thigh of your standing leg. Keep your pelvis in a neutral position. Lengthen your tailbone to the floor. Firmly press against the inner thigh of your standing leg with the foot of your bent leg, while resisting the pressure with your standing leg. Focus on a point in front of you to aid your balance. Hold for 30 seconds.

Be safe

Only lift your leg as high as feels comfortable.

DOWNWARD-FACING DOG (*right*)
AREAS TRAINED: SHOULDERS, ARMS, REAR THIGHS, CALVES

Technique

Kneel on the floor and place your hands shoulder-width apart on the floor. Lift your knees off the floor, pushing your sitting bones up to the ceiling and elongating your spine. Press your heels into the floor if you can. Don't force it. Contract your thighs and try to straighten your legs. Position your head in between your arms. Hold for 30 seconds to 2 minutes, elongating your spine.

Be safe

Don't over-stretch, and take extra care if you have high blood pressure.

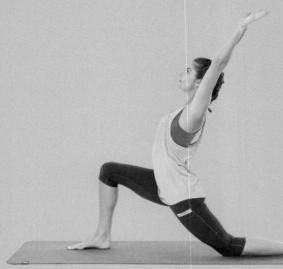

LOW LUNGE POSE *(left)*
AREAS TRAINED: FRONT THIGHS, HIPS, STOMACH

Technique

Start in a downward-facing dog position. Step one leg forward and place it in between your hands. Lower the knee of your back leg to the floor and rest the top of your left foot on the floor. Inhale and lift your torso to an upright position. Extend your arms up toward the ceiling. Lift your head upwards. Hold for 1 minute. Return to the downward-facing dog and repeat with the other leg.

Be safe

If your back knee hurts, place a towel under your knee.

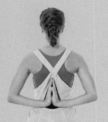

INTENSE SIDE STRETCH *(right)*
AREAS TRAINED: SHOULDERS, DEEP BACK MUSCLES, BOTTOM, REAR THIGHS, CALVES

Technique

Standing with your feet together, place your hands behind your back in a reverse prayer position. Step forward with one leg approximately 1–1.2 m (3–4 ft) forward. Turn your back foot out slightly while keeping your front foot pointing forward. Square your hips by pushing the hip bone of your back leg slightly forward. Press your back heel into the floor and contract your leg muscles. Lengthen your spine and lean forward with your spine. Keep your back flat, parallel with the floor. If you can, draw your torso down toward your front leg. Hold for 30 seconds. Repeat on the other side.

Be safe

Don't lift your back heel off the floor or round your back. Don't turn your hip out to either side.

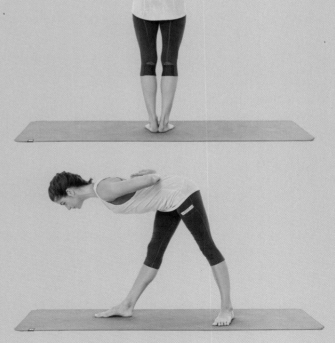

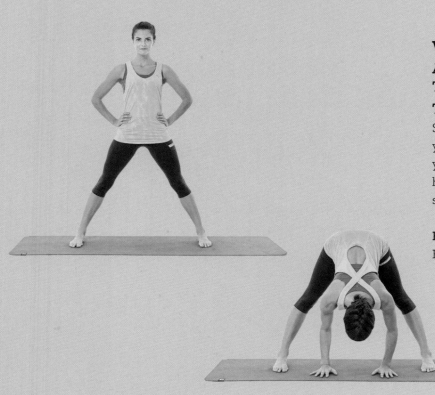

WIDE-LEGGED FORWARD BEND (left)
AREAS TRAINED: BOTTOM, REAR THIGHS, INNER THIGHS, DEEP BACK MUSCLES

Technique
Stand with your feet approximately 1–1.2 m (3–4 ft) apart. Keep your feet parallel to each other. Lengthen your spine and contract your stomach muscles. Bend forward from your hips. Place your hands on the floor in line with your shoulders. Keep your back straight. Hold for 30 seconds to 1 minute.

Be safe
Be careful if you have lower back issues.

COBRA POSE (right)
AREAS TRAINED: DEEP BACK MUSCLES, BOTTOM, CHEST, STOMACH, SHOULDERS

Technique
Lie on your stomach on the floor. Bend your elbows and place your hands flat on the floor next to your chest. Push your pubic bone, thighs, and the top of your feet into the floor. Lift your chest up, pushing your hands into the floor. Push your shoulders down and back, and elongate your neck while looking up slightly. Hold for 15–30 seconds.

Be safe
Take care if you have back problems. Only lift yourself up within a comfortable range of motion.

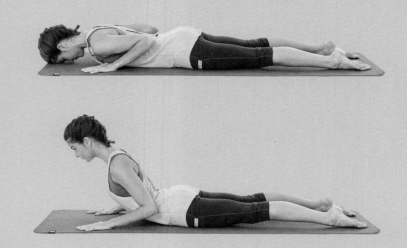

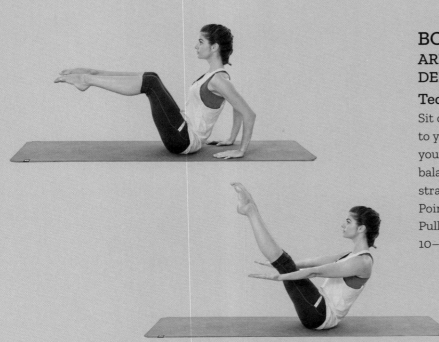

BOAT POSE *(left)*
AREAS TRAINED: STOMACH, SIDE MUSCLES, HIPS, DEEP BACK MUSCLE

Technique

Sit on the floor with your legs extended and your hands next to your side, fingers pointing forward. Bend your knees and lift your feet off the floor, leaning back with your shoulders. Find the balance point between your sitting bones and your tailbone. Slowly straighten your legs to form a 45-degree angle with your body. Point your toes and lift your arms sideways, parallel to the floor. Pull your tummy muscles tight and elongate your spine. Hold for 10–20 seconds.

Be safe

Avoid rounding your spine and sinking into your lower back. If you're unable to balance with your legs straight, balance with your knees bent.

TWISTING CHAIR POSE *(right)*
AREAS TRAINED: STOMACH, SIDE MUSCLES, REAR THIGHS, BOTTOM, DEEP BACK MUSCLES

Technique

Stand upright with your feet together. Squat down and extend your arms up. Lean back so that your weight rests on your heels. Squeeze your legs together and bring your hands down to your chest, pressing your palms together. Twist toward one side, placing your elbow on the outside of your opposite thigh. Stay in the squat position, keeping your spine elongated. Look up to the ceiling. Hold for 30 seconds, then repeat on the other side.

Be safe

Don't tense your stomach muscles too much, as this will prevent you from twisting.

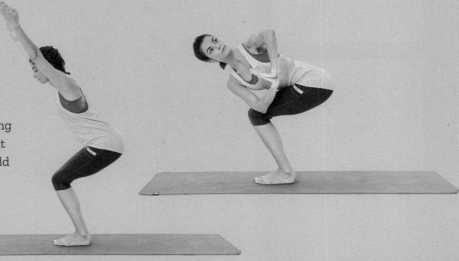

TIPS FOR A HEALTHY MENOPAUSE

Women usually begin going through the menopause around the age of 45–55. Periods become irregular and evenutally stop, but the transition affects each woman in a unique way. The following pages suggest ways of coping with some of the most common symptoms.

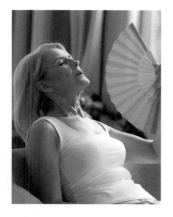

There are many symptoms of menopause, some relating to mental health and some physical. The first sign that menoapause is on its way (during the stage known as perimenopause) is usually a change in the normal pattern of your periods, for example they become irregular. Here's what else can happen:

- Changes to your mood, such as low mood, anxiety, mood swings, and low self-esteem.
- Problems with memory or concentration, sometimes called "brain fog."
- Hot flushes—a sudden temperature increase in your face, neck, and chest.
- Night sweats and difficulty sleeping, making you feel tired and irritable during the day.
- Palpitations, when you suddenly notice the feeing of your heart beating.
- Headaches and migraines.
- Muscle aches and joint pains.
- Weight gain or a change in your body shape.
- Skin changes, including dry and itchy skin.
- Reduced sex drive.
- Vaginal dryness, pain or itchiness, with discomfort during sex.
- Recurrent urinary tract infections (UTIs).

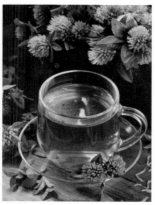

Here are some practical hints and tips that can help ease the symptoms of menopause and make you feel better in body and mind. **Note:** See your doctor if you are concerned about any of your symptoms or would like advice on medical interventions such as hormone replacment therapy (HRT).

SEEK HELP FROM HERBS
Soy and red clover provide plant estrogens that help reduce bouts of overheating. Sage is also thought to assist by curbing excessive sweating. Black cohosh could benefit you by balancing your hormones, but it isn't recommended if you have liver problems. Agnus cestus stabilizes hormones, too, and many women find it treats mood swings, anxiety, and tension. St John's wort may cut the number and severity of hot flushes and night sweats, and improve low mood. **Note:** If you are on any medication, check with your doctor before taking St John's wort, as it can react with some drugs.

FOCUS ON HEALTHY FATS

Not all fats are bad news—in fact, we need to include the right ones in our diet to support our body's functions and stay healthy. Polyunsaturated fats are needed for healthy brain functioning and are anti-inflammatory, which means they may reduce aches and pains and headaches. They are found in nuts and seeds, egg yolks, oily fish, and dark green leafy vegetables. Monounsaturated fats are rich in vitamin E and may promote hormonal balance. Red meat, full-fat milk, nuts, olives, olive and rapeseed oil, and avocados are good sources. Both types of fat can help to lower your cholesterol and reduce your risk of heart disease.

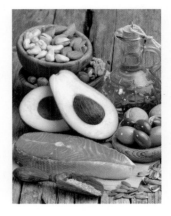

DRINK CRANBERRY JUICE

To help prevent cystitis, which affects some women at menopause, wear cotton underwear. Synthetic fibers trap moisture and bacteria. If you suffer from recurrent cystitis, drink cranberry juice twice daily—evidence suggests it can reduce the number of infections, as cranberries contain substances that discourage bacteria from sticking to the bladder and urethra. If you do get cystitis, drink a tumbler of water with 1 teaspoon of bicarbonate of soda three times a day to help make your urine less acidic. **Note:** If symptoms worsen, see your doctor.

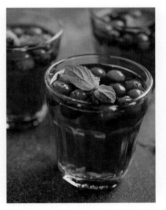

CUT DOWN ON TEA AND COFFEE

Both the temperature of a cup of tea or coffee and the stimulant effects of the caffeine they contain can trigger hot flushes. The amount of caffeine in a cup varies according to the strength of the brand, the amount used, and brewing time, so bear these factors in mind if you can't do without your caffeine fix. You can curb your intake by replacing a few cups each day with decaffeinated tea or coffee, or a herbal tea, such as Rooibos or chamomile, which has soothing, sedative effects, making it the perfect bedtime drink. Cold water is another obvious choice to help you avoid overheating. You can make it even more cooling and refreshing by adding mint, or slices of lemon or cucumber, and chilling it in the fridge before drinking.

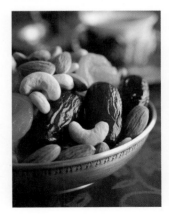

BORON!

Boron is a less-well-known mineral that can help menopausal symptoms. It has been found to boost estrogen and help the body absorb calcium and magnesium, helping to prevent osteoporosis and aches and pains. It's found naturally in fruit (especially apples, oranges, pears, avocados, red grapes, dried apricots, dates, and prunes), vegetables (greens, broccoli, carrots, celery, and potatoes), pulses or legumes (kidney beans, lentils, and chickpeas) and nuts (almonds, Brazil nuts, cashew nuts, hazelnuts, peanuts, and walnuts).

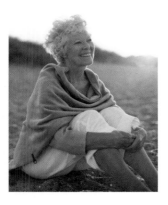

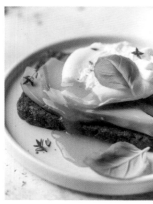

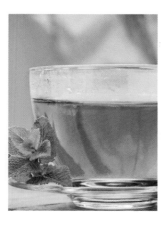

SOAK UP A LITTLE SUN

If you suffer from low moods, you may find that dull, rainy weather can make you feel even more miserable. So when the sun does shine, it's vital to take advantage of the mood boost and other health benefits it offers. Exposure to the sun's rays kick-starts our skin cells into making vitamin D, which helps the brain to produce serotonin, our "happy hormone." Short, daily spells of direct sunlight on the skin—around 10–15 minutes—can give us the vitamin D we need to boost mood and energy levels; after this you should apply sun cream to avoid sun damage. You'll benefit even on cloudy days, though it takes the body a little longer to produce the vitamin without direct sunlight.

POWER UP WITH PROTEIN

Eating protein at each meal helps you manage your weight because protein takes longer to digest, thereby keeping you fuller for longer. There's evidence that people who eat a high-protein breakfast, such as poached or boiled eggs on whole wheat (wholemeal) toast, tend to eat less during the rest of the day. The body uses protein to build muscle, and muscle will rev up your metabolism, which in turn helps prevent middle-aged spread. Eggs, lean meat, fish, beans, and legumes are all good sources of protein. Choose a healthy cooking method, such as boiling, steaming, poaching, grilling, or baking.

BEAT THE BLOAT

While bloating at menopause is linked to hormonal changes, modifying your eating habits should bring some relief. Although fiber helps digestion, insoluble fiber found in wholegrains can ferment in the gut, causing wind. If you're affected, choose foods containing soluble fiber, which is gentler on the stomach (porridge oats, oat cakes, and oatbread). Likewise, avoid beans, peas, cabbage, sprouts, and onions if you notice they give you wind. Excess salt encourages water retention, so avoid salty snacks and don't add salt to meals. Seasoning food with black pepper can help the body break it down, reducing bloating, while drinking ginger or peppermint tea after a meal can aid digestion and release trapped wind. Fizzy drinks are full of gas, so it may be wise to ditch them. Finally, relax and enjoy your food—gulping it down means you're swallowing air, which leads to bloating.

SPARE THE SUGAR

Eating too much sugar is linked to a litany of health woes, including weight gain, type 2 diabetes, heart disease, and stroke, as well as dental problems and aging skin. Refined sugary foods lead to a sharp rise in blood sugar, which then falls just as fast, leaving you hungry and craving more sugar. Low blood sugar may also trigger a hot flush. Keep processed foods with added sugar to a minimum. Instead, base your meals on proteins, wholegrains, fruit and vegetables, nuts and seeds, and healthy fats.

EXERCISE TO EASE STRESS

If you're feeling anxious or stressed, or are suffering from hot flushes, working out may be the furthest thing from your mind. But studies show that women who exercise during the menopause report a more positive mood and better sense of wellbeing. Exercise encourages the release of mood-boosting serotonin and endorphins. Any activity that involves repetitive movements can produce the same effect, such as cycling, taking a brisk walk, swimming, or rowing.

STAY HYDRATED

Drinking sufficient water is always important, whatever your age, but even more so during menopause, when good hydration can help prevent the development of other health issues such as cystitis and migraines. It's especially important to replace the fluid lost through hot flushes and night sweats. Experts recommend we drink at least 1.2 liters or 6–8 large glasses of fluid a day—although in hot weather you may need more. This can include tea and coffee in moderation. You also get water from the food you eat, including fruits (such as watermelon, oranges, and apples), vegetables (such as cucumbers, tomatoes, and iceberg lettuce), soups, and broths. These foods can give you around a fifth of your total fluid intake.

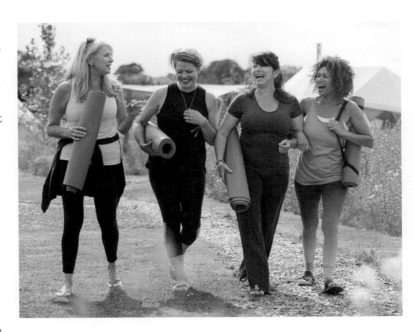

FEEL COOLER WITH THIS MIND TRICK!

Visualizing being in a cool place has been shown to help reduce hot flushes. For example, imagine being outside on a freezing cold day, or lowering yourself into an ice-cold plunge pool. Feel the sensation of coldness slowly spreading up throughout your body from your toes to the top of your head. Other mental images that have been shown to help combat flushes include picturing standing beneath a waterfall or rain shower, feeling cool air or a cool breeze on the skin, or being in a forest.

ENJOY "ME TIME"

Life gets busy, so it's important to take time out to relax. Perhaps you could spend an evening curled up with a good book or watching your favorite TV show, indulge in a long soak in a warm, scented bath, or simply find time for a hobby you enjoy and appreciate being in your own company.

FEED YOUR BONES AND JOINTS

Women can lose as much as 20 percent of their bone mass during menopause, which is a startling statistic. This can result in osteoporosis, with the bones breaking more easily. So it's very important for women to choose foods that strengthen their bones and joints as they get older.

PROTECTING YOUR BONES

Oestrogen production in women slows down in the middle years, and there are certain well-documented symptoms that may be experienced: disrupted sleep, hot flashes, and mood swings, to name but three. But one of the hidden effects of those changing hormones is the depletion of bone density. You can help protect against this by looking at the foods you eat and making sure they're giving you an adequate intake of calcium and vitamin D, both of which help to build strong bones.

- For calcium, eat plenty of green leafy vegetables, fermented soya products, nuts, and oily fish. Most of these are also rich in protein, which studies have shown is critical for maintaining bone density.
- Vitamin D is a key nutrient that helps you absorb calcium. The body's ability to produce vitamin D from exposure to sunlight decreases with age and it can be difficult to get enough from your diet, so supplementation is a good idea. Food-based sources include oily fish, eggs, and fortified products.

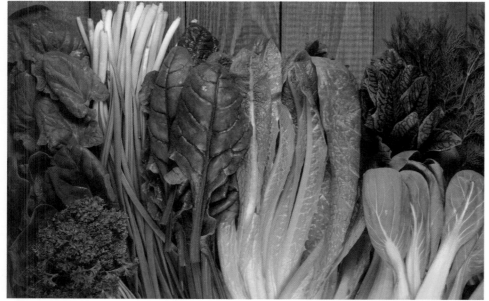

EASING YOUR JOINTS

It's not just bones that take a hit in midlife. Another symptom of the menopause is joint pain, and arthritis can also be a concern. Eating more anti-inflammatory foods and good healthy fats may help—so make sure you're eating nuts and seeds, broccoli, cauliflower, kale, ginger, turmeric, oily fish and extra virgin olive oil, which are all joint-friendly foods.

Note: There's lots you can eat in midlife to support your bone and joint health, but if you are experiencing any symptoms or have a family history of osteoporosis or arthritis, it's worth having a chat about it with your doctor.

TOP 3 FOODS FOR BONE AND JOINT HEALTH

To build and protect your bones and joints, it would help to include these three foods in your diet:

1. Natural yogurt

Natural, unsweetened yogurt has plenty of calcium, and if you can find one that's fortified with vitamin D, you'll get even more bone health benefits. Stir it into porridge, soups, curries, and stews. It's also a healthier alternative to mayonnaise in dips and spreads.

2. Tinned sardines

Oily fish are brilliant for joints, and sardines are an excellent source of calcium, too. Try combining tinned sardines (in extra virgin olive oil) with red onion, chopped flat-leaf parsley, olives, lemon juice, and a dash of tabasco for an excellent toast topping.

3. Chia seeds

Rich in calcium and ALAs (a type of anti-inflammatory omega-3 fatty acid), chia seeds are a great addition to your diet. Make a simple chia pudding by combining the seeds with milk and refrigerating overnight, or make chia jam by mixing the seeds with mashed fresh fruit.

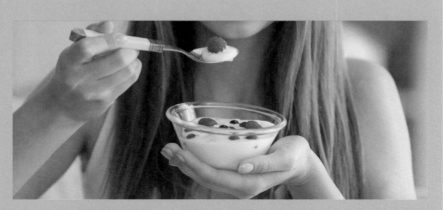

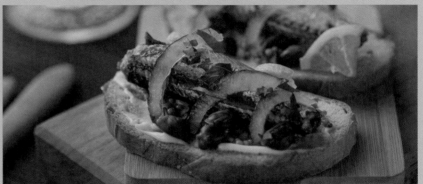

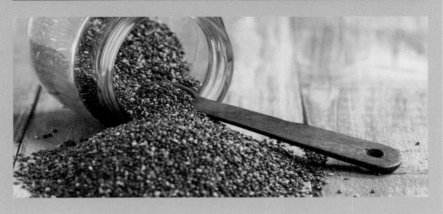

HEALTH TIPS FOR OLDER MEN

Generally speaking, the average man probably pays less attention to his health than the average woman. However, the aging process affects everyone, and there are certain areas when older men need to take extra care.

30 MINUTES A DAY

It is recommended that older adults do at least 30 minutes of moderate exercise every day. But if that seems too much, note that *some* activity is always better than none—even if it's just strolling around the block or pottering in the garden for half an hour.

Men can be affected by many of the same diseases as women — such as heart disease, stroke, diabetes, cancer, and depression—but they have their own unique issues, too, such as prostate cancer, testicular cancer, erectile dysfunction, and low testosterone. They are also more likely to drink alcohol, smoke, make risky choices, and avoid visiting their doctor to ask for help. Many of the major health risks that men face can be reduced by living a healthy lifestyle.

REGULAR EXERCISE

Choose a form of exercise that corresponds to your personal level of fitness. Most older men should aim to do some moderate aerobic exercise, such as brisk walking, cycling, and swimming, while fitter men could add more vigorous activities such jogging, running, or hill walking. Golf is another excellent choice—it's been claimed that golf can extend your life by five years! It improves cardiovascular fitness, reduces the risk of chronic conditions, improves your strength and balance, and provides a positive social life at the same time. Bodyweight exercises, such as squats, push-ups, and step-ups, are also a good idea. They will help to increase muscle tone, maintain strength, build bone density, keep you at a healthy weight, optimize metabolic function, and reduce the risk of injury, falls, and fatigue.

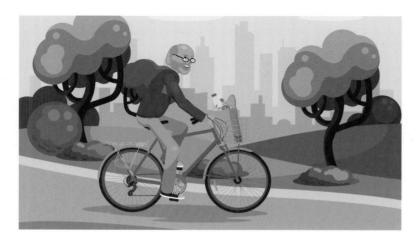

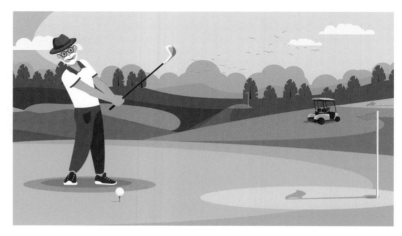

HEALTHY DIET

It goes without saying that older men should eat a healthy diet, and in addition to this, it's also a good idea to limit drinking to within the moderate range—which means no more than two drinks a day, if that. Reducing alcohol consumption not only means you'll lose weight, have more energy, and feel healthier overall, you'll also be reducing your risk of developing long-term health problems such as heart disease, cancer, or cirrhosis (scarring) of the liver.

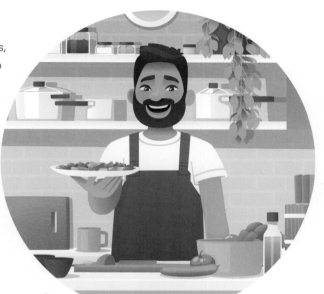

QUIT SMOKING

Being cigarette-free significantly reduces the risk of cardiovascular disease, chronic obstructive pulmonary disease (COPD), lung and throat cancer, emphysema, high blood pressure, ulcers and reflux, erectile and sexual dysfunction, and kidney disease, and can add as much as 10 years to your life expectancy.

REDUCE YOUR STRESS

A study published in the July 2000 issue of *Psychological Review* stated that although men and women are both exposed to stress, they handle it differently. Essentially, the hormonal differences between the two genders accounts for the different responses—men produce less oxytocin than women, which causes men to have a stronger "fight-or-flight" response. This explains why so many men either bottle up their problems or seek ways to escape them altogether. In any case, stress leads to an increase in blood pressure, raised blood sugar levels, and a weaker immune system, and when left untreated can result in serious health problems. So, if you find yourself stressing out over a problem or worrying at night to the point where you're not sleeping, try the following:

- Regular physical activities.
- Relaxation techniques, such as deep breathing, meditation, yoga, or tai chi.
- Socialize with your family and friends.
- Spend time on your hobbies or other recreational activities.
- Talk to a health professional.

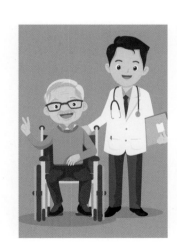

MEDICAL CHECKUPS

As we get older, regular checkups are always a good idea. Your doctor can check your blood pressure, cholesterol, and heart health, and also make sure you're a healthy weight. Older men, in particular, need to attend regular screening tests for conditions such as prostate cancer and bowel cancer. The tests can detect these diseases early when they're much easier to treat, so it's always best to set aside any embarrassment and put your health needs first.

AVOID DEMENTIA

Dementia is a general term for the impaired ability to remember, think or make decisions, and although it tends to occur in older people, it is not a normal part of the aging process. Here, one of the world's top brain surgeons, Dr. Rahul Jandial, gives his lifestyle tips for keeping your mind and memory sharp well into old age.

GET ENOUGH SLEEP

For Dr. Jandial, the brain is inextricably linked to mood and emotions, and one of the things that can affect both is sleep. "We know [prolonged] lack of sleep affects everything. It can cause heart disease and other metabolic issues and is linked with mental health issues and Alzheimer's. But another thing people don't often talk about is how it can change your mood and emotional regulation," says Dr. Jandial. "You're more sensitive, grumpy, and more likely to feel hurt... People with dementia don't just get lost and forget things. They're frustrated, upset, emotional, labile. Mood and memory are linked."

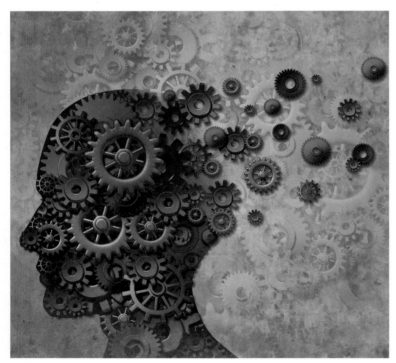

LET THERE BE (LESS) LIGHT

"The rotation of the earth, switching from dark to light, affects everything on the planet, from plants to animals to us, and the most important thing about sleep is light management," says Dr. Jandial. Traditionally, dimming daylight would signal to your brain to start winding down, preparing you for slumber. But with so much artificial light in our environments now, many people are out of synch with natural light-dark cycles. "The simplest advice is to start dimming the lights around 7–8 pm. That will set off the natural triggers to initiate sleep," he says. This includes the lighting in your home, as well as your TV, laptop screens, and phones.

BREATHE DEEPLY

Do your thoughts keep wandering when you try to meditate? It turns out that's OK, as it's your breathing that's the most important factor. This has been studied through experiments involving opening people's skulls and inserting grids on their brains, giving researchers a "live feed" of activity! 'When asked to do controlled deep breathing—3 seconds in, hold, 3 seconds out—the researchers found that regardless of what the participants were thinking, it changed the electrical flows within those people's brains," says Dr. Jandial. "Controlled breathing is your built-in tranquility mode, triggering the release of chemicals that have an instant calming effect." It's something he recommends weaving into everyday life. "Whether that's five minutes before you get home because you're frustrated, or five minutes because you've been fighting with your partner, these results happen within minutes—you don't need hours, or to go to a silent retreat."

TRAIN YOUR BRAIN

Memory is often described as a muscle that can be trained—so does this mean reliance on modern technology is harming our future brain health? Dr. Jandial doesn't think it's as simplistic as that. Plus, some types of memory do naturally decrease with age—such as the ability to remember names and where you put your keys. "Our phones are going to help us with those things, they're our allies," he says. But there's plenty you can do to "train" your memory and help stay sharp. "Your frontal lobe is excellent at what's called 'working memory' or as I prefer to call it, the 'multi-tasking' or 'juggling memory.' This is the one we all ought to work on," he says. Although multi-tasking gets a bad rap, Dr. Jandial says it's how effectively you do it that counts and that mental juggling—without dropping any balls—is the best kind of memory practice there is. You can also weave training tricks into your day-to-day routine. "For example, try to remember what's on your calendar or to-do list before you look at it. Or look at your route before setting off somewhere, then see how far you can get without having to check the map again. That's the memory that's going to keep you effective at work and life."

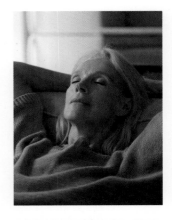

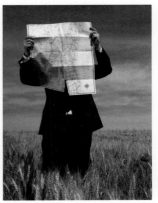

MOVE YOUR BODY

Exercise has endless benefits for the brain, starting with simply keeping up its vital blood supply. "The brain is flesh and needs to be irrigated as much as any other part of the body—more than other parts of the body, in fact, because it's only 5 kg (11 lb) but gets 20 percent of the body's blood flow. It's an energy hog!" And if you have clogged arteries, you'll have swathes of brain wither inside your skull. This is essentially what happens with vascular dementia, which occurs due to restricted blood flow to the brain. "Physical activity also enables you to activate your own 'internal pharmacy'," says Dr. Jandial, triggering the release of feel-good chemicals including dopamine and serotonin, which play a huge role in mental health. And it doesn't actually take much exercise to reap the benefits. "These [chemicals] are not only released if you become a marathon runner. They're released if you simply go from sitting around to standing and walking more," he says. "Regularly going for brisk 30-minute daily walks has been found to provide around an 80 percent health boost from these feel-good chemicals, while super fitness fanatics may be getting 90 percent." It's time to lace up those walking boots!

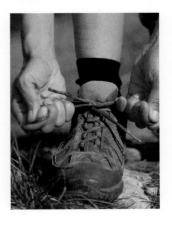

PLANNERS

The following pages contain some planners to help you devise daily routines that work specifically for you—whether it be your work/life balance, your exercise routine, or your food consumption. There are also pages for you to write notes and jot down your thoughts about how you achieve your optimum lifestyle.

ROUTINE PLANNER

Use this planner to devise a daily and weekly routine that works for you.

TIME \ DAY	MONDAY	TUESDAY	WEDNESDAY
6.00am			
7.00am			
8.00am			
9.00am			
10.00am			
11.00am			
12.00pm			
1.00pm			
2.00pm			
3.00pm			
4.00pm			
5.00pm			
6.00pm			
7.00pm			
8.00pm			
9.00pm			
10.00pm			
11.00pm			

THURSDAY	FRIDAY	SATURDAY	SUNDAY

EXERCISE AND ACTIVITY PLANNER

Use this planner to record your daily exercise or activities that you enjoy.

MONDAY	TUESDAY	WEDNESDAY
DAY	DAY	DAY
EVENING	EVENING	EVENING

THURSDAY	FRIDAY	SATURDAY	SUNDAY
DAY	DAY	DAY	DAY
EVENING	EVENING	EVENING	EVENING

FOOD PLANNER

Use this planner to keep a food diary or work out your meals for the week.

MEAL \ DAY	MONDAY	TUESDAY	WEDNESDAY
Breakfast			
Mid-morning			
Lunch			
Mid-Afternoon			
Dinner			

THURSDAY	FRIDAY	SATURDAY	SUNDAY

NOTES

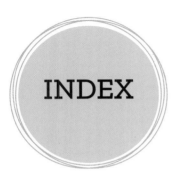

INDEX

'ABC' approach **62**
Aesop **84**
ageing
    attitude to **210–11**
    dementia **244–5**
    diet for **119–21**, **221**, **241**, **243**
    exercise **211**, **220**, **222–35**, **242**, **245**
    gardening **226–7**
    menopause **223**, **236–9**
    men's health **242–3**
    mitochondria **228–9**
    osteoporosis **240–1**
    running **224–5**
    spirit age **212–15**
    staying young **218–21**
    stress reduction **216–17**, **239**, **243**
    women's health **223**, **236–9**, **240–1**
    yoga **230–5**
alcohol **83**, **101**
Allen, Chris **138**, **139**
alternative therapies **204**
anxiety **52–3**, **78**
Archer, Jeff **47**
Aria, Dr **51**, **57**

arm exercises **150–1**
Arroll, Megan **30**, **31**, **51**, **56**

back pain **174–5**
bedtime routine **196**
behaviour understanding **81**
Benoit Samuelson, Joan **225**
Bhajan, Yogi **158**
Bond, Tim **63**, **64**
Bose, Simone **34**
Bostock, Richie **22**, **23**
boundaries **26**
Boyce, Carol **44**, **46**
brain boosts **170–1**
breakfasts **19**, **201**
breathing techniques
    ageing **244–5**
    energy boosting **203**
    lifestyle **22–5**
    mental health **75**
    sleep **196**
Brewer, Sarah **179**
Brinkley, Christie **212**
Brocksopp, Lorna **84**, **85**, **87**

caffeine **20**, **65**, **83**, **229**
Callenberg, Amanda **65**
career development **36–42**
Carr, Lucie **86**
Chamberlain, Steve **200**, **201**
Charman, Hannah **177**
Chatterjee, Rangan **114**
choirs **29**
Choudhury, Bikram **157**

Clark, Laura **112**
Cohen, Sheldon **31**, **32**
colds **176–7**
complementary therapies **204**
cortisol **181**
Coventry, John **85**
Crew, Alastair **143**
Cullen, Alison **61**, **216**, **217**
cycling **140–1**

Dahl, Cortland **63**, **64**
Dale, Claire **22**, **23**
De-Lisser, Mark **171**
decluttering **14–17**
dementia **244–5**
depression **71–5**
diet
    ageing **119–21**, **241**, **243**
    energy boost **206–7**
    fibre **104–5**
    fluids **98–9**
    food groups **94–5**
    gut health **112–15**
    happiness **116**
    heart health **106–7**
    immune system **100–1**
    libido **118**
    and mental health **65**, **72**
    protein **102–3**
    recipes **128–9**
    sleep **196**, **197**
    stress reduction **108–11**, **117**

and type **2** diabetes **181–3**
    veganism **96–7**
    vegetarianism **96–7**
    weight loss **122–9**
digital decluttering **15**
dopamine fasting **82–3**

energy levels
    boosting **202–3**, **205–7**
    mental health **63–5**
environmental action **168–9**
exercise
    and ageing **211**, **220**, **222–35**, **242**, **245**
    for arms **150–1**
    cycling **140–1**
    enjoyment of **132–5**
    equipment for **144–5**
    15-minute workout **146–8**
    fitting in **149**
    for glutes **152–5**
    heart health **138–9**
    intuitive fitness **136–7**
    and mental health **57**, **66–7**, **72**
    pilates **160**
    7-day plan for **162–3**
    sports **161**
    stretching **142–3**
    and type 2 diabetes **180**
    yoga **156–9**

fats **181**
fibre **104**–**5**
15-minute workout **146**–**8**
Fisher, Maggie **188**
fluids **98**–**9**, **220**
food groups **94**–**5**
Ford, Henry **45**
friendships **30**–**3**, **211**
forest bathing **11**, **18**, **76**–**7**

Gabe-Thomas, Lizzi **18**
Gannon, Sharon **158**
gardening **226**–**7**
Georgiou, Katerina **33**
Gibson, Glenn **115**
glutes exercises **152**–**5**
goal-setting **44**–**7**
Good Thinking
  programme **56**
Goodwin, Holly **136**, **137**
gratitude **46**, **54**, **57**, **90**
Gratton, Lynda **210**
Greenberg, David **20**
gut health **112**–**15**

hairstyles **219**
happiness **116**
heart health
  diet **106**–**7**
  exercise **138**–**9**
  sleep **191**
herbs **174**, **236**
high-intensity interval
  training (HIIT) **229**

Hildegard of Bingen **207**
hugs **31**

immune system **100**–**1**, **191**
intuitive fitness **136**–**7**
Iyengar, B.K.S. **157**

James, Margareta **50**
Jandial, Rahul **244**, **245**
journal keeping **46**

Kaia app **175**
Katus, Hugo **186**
Kellett, Jo **198**
Khan, Tahira **173**
kindness **84**–**7**

Lamb, Fiona **170**
libido **118**
Life, David **158**
lifestyle
  boundaries **26**
  breathing techniques
    22–**5**
  career development
    36–**42**
  changes in **27**
  decluttering **14**–**17**
  friendships **30**–**3**
  goal-setting **44**–**7**
  nature fixes **18**
  questions about **9**
  relationship break-ups
    34–**5**

routines **19**–**21**
  stress reduction **28**–**9**
  work/life balance **41**, **43**,
    46
Lockwood, Rebecca **173**
loneliness **70**

Marogy, Aliza **65**
massage **75**, **173**, **205**
Maubec, Sheila **230**, **231**
McConville, Stephen **138**
McIntosh, Diane **71**
McKenna, Sarah **219**
meditation **21**, **74**
Mehl, Konstantin **175**
menopause **223**, **236**–**9**
men's health **186**–**7**, **242**–**3**
mental health
  anxiety **52**–**3**
  behaviour
    understanding **81**
  categories in **78**
  depression **71**–**5**
  dopamine fasting **82**–**3**
  forest bathing **76**–**7**
  kindness **84**–**7**
  loneliness **70**
  negative thinking **58**–**9**,
    80
  stress reduction **60**–**9**
  talking **73**, **79**
  worrying **50**–**1**, **54**–**7**
Middleton, Nick **174**
migraines **172**–**3**

Miller, Michael Craig **72**
mindful breathing **25**
mindfulness **89**
mitochondria **228**–**9**
Mohidin, Roshane **66**
Moore, Alison **213**, **214**, **215**
Morgan, Kim **43**
Moulton, Vanessa **33**
multi-tasking **59**
music **21**, **74**, **83**

natural light **65**, **74**
nature fixes **18**, **29**, **72**
Neal, Christina **58**
Neff, Kristin **91**
negative thinking **58**–**9**, **80**
Neurolinguistic
  programming (NLP) **173**

oils **174**
osteopathy **175**
osteoporosis **240**–**1**

paced breathing **25**
Panagos, Angelique **116**
parenting **188**–**9**
pets **28**, **73**, **218**
physical wellbeing
  alternative therapies
    204
  back pain **174**–**5**
  benefits of **11**
  brain boosts **170**–**1**
  colds **176**–**7**

complementary
  therapies 204
energy boosters 202–3,
  205–7
environmental action
  168–9
men's health 186–7
migraines 172–3
parenting 188–9
sleep 170, 179, 181,
  190–201
spiritual self–care 166–7
type 2 diabetes 180–3
virus-prevention 178–9
women's health 184–5
pilates 160
Pitchiah, Balu 50, 51
pranayama 25
protein 102–3, 182, 238

Ramsden, Natalia 82, 83
relationship break–ups
  34–5
relaxation 69
Rescue Remedy 50
Robinson, Rebecca 225
routines 19–21, 75
running 224–5

Salcedas, Christina 199
Sathyapala, Amanda 228,
  229
Schweet, Carley 166
Scott, Andrew 210

self-compassion 88–91
Sepah, Cameron 82, 83
7-day exercise plan 162–3
singing 171
Singh, Reenee 79
Sivananda, Swami 158
sleep
  and ageing 218, 244
  bedtime routine 196
  diet 196, 197
  importance of 190–1
  improving 192–5
  and mental health 61
  and physical well-being
    170, 179, 181, 190–201
  smells for 198–9
  waking up 200–1
smells 28, 198–9
spirit age 212–15
spiritual self–care 166–7
Spock, Benjamin 189
sports 161
Steinhilber, Brianna 90
stress reduction
  ageing 216–17, 239, 243
  diet 18–11, 117
  lifestyle 28–9
  mental health 60–9
stretching 142–3, 200
supplements 55, 65, 183
Swift, Hannah 212, 214, 215
swimming 73

Taikyu, Sandy 202

Talking 73, 79
Tatum, Mary K. 71
Thurner, Manuel 175
type 2 diabetes 180–3

veganism 96–7
vegetarianism 96–7
virus-prevention 178–9

waking up 200–1
Ward, Karol 50, 51
water 98–9, 200
Watkins, Alan 51
weight control 122–9, 223
Whyte, Greg 160
Wiener, David 67
Wilk, Anna 44, 45
Williams, Charlie 86
Williams, Lucia 44
women's health 184–5, 223,
  236–9, 240–1
work/life balance 41, 43, 46
worrying 50–1, 54–7

yoga
  ageing 230–5
  as exercise 156–9
  mental health 68–9